Advance Praise for *The Non-Toxic Aven*

Deanna Duke provides wonderful insights in this very personal exploration of the toxic chemicals hidden in every single part of our lives. An important and timely guide to understanding our toxic world.

— Bruce Lourie, co-author *Slow Death by Rubber Duck*

In *The Non-Toxic Avenger*, Deanna Duke lays out what could otherwise be confusing information in a straightforward, non-hysterical, and relatable way. The beauty of this book is that readers can apply Deanna's nontoxic avenging in small or large ways, taking as tiny or as enormous a step as they like. Either way, it will make readers think a little harder about the things we humans surround, slather, coat, and feed ourselves with. It was an eye-opener for me.

— Ree Drummond, ThePioneerWoman.com,
author of *The Pioneer Woman Cooks* and host,
The Pioneer Woman cooking show (Food Network)

There are a lot of things in this book you probably think you'd rather not know. Not knowing, however, doesn't reduce your risk or improve your life. Deanna Duke is brave enough to want to know, and wise enough to give us the information we truly need in a way that enriches. This is an important, funny, wonderful and courageous book that you truly do want to read.

— Sharon Astyk, author, *Depletion and Abundance*
and *Independence Days* and science writer at www.sharonastyk.com

Wow! That's the only way to describe Deanna Duke's heart-stopping, eye-popping, head-shaking quest to figure out what toxic chemicals threaten not only her life and the lives of the people she loves, but the lives of each and every one of us as well. Start this book and don't stop until you're done. Yes, you'll cry. But you'll also laugh. And then, hopefully, you'll get busy — clearing out your cupboards, writing to your elected officials, and telling everyone you know that they MUST read this incredible, courageous, inspiring book, too.

— Diane MacEachern, author, *Big Green Purse: Use Your Spending Power to Create a Cleaner, Greener World*
and founder, www.biggreenpurse.com.

Duke offers a revealing look at the dangers lurking within our clothing, food, and household products—her personal battle against these is at once deeply moving and totally hilarious.

— Vanessa Farquharson, author, *Sleeping Naked is Green*

The idea that our home environment and product choices can make us sick is a powerful motivator for cleaner living. *The Non-Toxic Avenger* is the perfect guide for anyone seeking to lower their toxic body burden and protect their families.

— Tiffany Washko, blogger, naturemoms.com

The Non-Toxic Avenger is not a hard-core prescription against toxic chemicals, but rather an insightful (and humorous!) look into the challenges of "clean" living in a world without meaningful chemical regulations.

— Micaela Preston, author, *Practically Green:
Your Guide to EcoFriendly Decision-Making*,
and blogger, MindfulMomma.typepad.com

Author Deanna Duke leads us through her journey with refreshing honesty, admitting her own hypochondriac tendencies and imperfections. With the help of body burden testing and a team of forward-thinking experts, she finds clues about what happens when simple steps are taken to decrease some of the biggest offending chemicals like BPA, flame retardants and triclosan. And most importantly, Deanna gives credence to the notion that you really can improve your health when armed with the right information and some stick-to-it determination.

— Alicia Voorhies, RN, founder, TheSoftLanding.com

THE NON-TOXIC AVENGER

WHAT YOU DON'T KNOW CAN HURT YOU

DEANNA DUKE

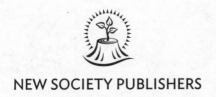

NEW SOCIETY PUBLISHERS

Cover design by Diane McIntosh.

Printed in Canada. First printing September 2011.

Paperback ISBN: 978-0-86571-692-6
eISBN: 978-1-55092-486-2

Inquiries regarding requests to reprint all or part of *The Non-Toxic Avenger*
should be addressed to New Society Publishers at the address below.

To order directly from the publishers, please call toll-free (North America)
1-800-567-6772, or order online at www.newsociety.com

Any other inquiries can be directed by mail to:

New Society Publishers
P.O. Box 189, Gabriola Island, BC V0R 1X0, Canada
(250) 247-9737

New Society Publishers' mission is to publish books that contribute in fundamental ways
to building an ecologically sustainable and just society, and to do so with the least possible
impact on the environment, in a manner that models this vision. We are committed to doing
this not just through education, but through action. The interior pages of our bound books
are printed on Forest Stewardship Council-registered acid-free paper that is **100% post-
consumer recycled** (100% old growth forest-free), processed chlorine free, and printed with
vegetable-based, low-VOC inks, with covers produced using FSC-registered stock. New
Society also works to reduce its carbon footprint, and purchases carbon offsets based on
an annual audit to ensure a carbon neutral footprint. For further information, or to browse
our full list of books and purchase securely, visit our website at: www.newsociety.com

LIBRARY AND ARCHIVES CANADA CATALOGUING IN PUBLICATION

Duke, Deanna
The non-toxic avenger : what you don't know can hurt you / Deanna Duke.

Includes index.
ISBN 978-0-86571-692-6

1. Environmental toxicology—Popular works.   2. Household supplies—Toxicology—
Popular works.   3. Product safety—Popular works.   I. Title.

RA1213.D86 2011   615.9'02   C2011-905922-3

NEW SOCIETY PUBLISHERS
www.newsociety.com

MIX
Paper from
responsible sources
FSC® C016245

Contents

Acknowledgments

First and foremost I would like to thank my family for tolerating my toxin paranoia and for letting me change a considerable number of products in their lives. Although these changes were for the better and will reduce their overall toxic burden, change is always difficult, particularly when you are asking someone to eliminate a favorite product or, worse, a favorite toy or piece of jewelry. So, in that vein I would like to thank my children, Henry and Emma, and my husband, Hank, who bore the brunt of most of my toxic fits.

I would also like to thank Sharon Astyk, Philip Rutter and Ron Coacher for being sounding boards and keeping me on track, and my mother for being responsive to my requests to stop bringing potentially toxic items and gifts into our household. Additionally, I would like to thank the readers of my blog who have been following my non-toxic journey and have given me feedback in many valuable ways.

This project could not have happened without the help of Dr. Steven Gilbert of Toxipedia and the Institute of Neurotoxicology & Neurological Disorders who provided a wealth of resources and review. I would also like to thank Erika Schreder, Staff Scientist at the Washington Toxics Coalition, for her guidance in getting body burden testing as well as providing a resource for XRF analysis. Finally, thanks to Dr. John Hibbs from Bastyr, who assisted in arranging the lab tests I underwent to determine my toxic body burden, and provided information on the impacts of environmental toxins and detoxing as well as on how to interpret the test results.

My never-ending thanks to those who had the fortitude to beta-read this book: Joseph Tisa, Steven Gilbert, Earl Krygier, Cynthia Hernandez, Lisa Coacher and Henry Daehnke.

Last but not least, I have to thank everyone at New Society Publishers for helping bring this book to fruition and letting me switch gears and pretty much do whatever the hell I wanted with this book.

PART

I

Laying It All Out

In the Beginning

I thought I lived a fairly clean lifestyle. I didn't use pesticides in my yard, tried to choose organic foods, stayed away from overly processed products and didn't smoke. What I *thought* was the whole shebang of avoiding toxins. But, like most people, I had my faults. I still used conventional cosmetics and some body and hair care products and I relied on the good old power of caustic cleaners. Since I lived a pretty focused life of trying to lower my carbon footprint, I thought that, by reducing my petroleum usage and generally choosing natural products, I was in the clear.

I firmly believed that if a product were sold on the shelves in the store, that product was safe to use unless it stated otherwise. Some of them may not have been the most environmentally friendly to use but they were safe. The FDA says so, doesn't it? And I was more than happy to put my faith in government agencies and turn a blind eye to the real story just to keep believing that those plastics in my mascara and the preservatives in my shampoo were innocuous and I could have silky hair and glowing skin in spite of what the ingredient labels did and did not tell me.

It wasn't until I received a review copy of the book *Slow Death by Rubber Duck: The Secret Danger of Everyday Things* for my environmental blog, *The Crunchy Chicken*, that I started to think otherwise. In the circle of individuals who were blogging on

1

environmental topics, there was always a subset that focused on toxins in products. I figured that was their bailiwick, not mine. I was more concerned with reducing waste, energy usage and the strain on the environment from personal carbon footprints. The closest I got to dealing with the topic on my blog was really in relation to issues with agriculture and its incumbent petroleum-based fertilizer and pesticide use. But that didn't matter to me personally because I didn't choose products produced by conventional agriculture. Or did it? Were the health problems my family faced a result of environmental toxins, bad genetics or both?

Double whammy

Since I started writing my blog and really focusing on environmental issues, two very personal things had happened. The first was that my son, Henry, was diagnosed with Asperger's syndrome, a mild form of autism. The second was that my husband, Hank, was diagnosed with multiple myeloma, an incurable, extremely life-shortening form of leukemia. Both were diagnosed the same week in September 2007. I still haven't recovered from it all but, then again, neither have they.

During the last six months of Henry's preschool year, in 2007, I would be filled with dread every time the phone rang. I was convinced that it was his preschool calling to tell me, yet again, that Henry had hit, kicked or, God forbid, bit another child. His school environment was more staid than the average preschool given that it was a Montessori school and a fairly rigid one at that. But it was far too stimulating for my son and, when it got overwhelming or when kids got too close or too much in his face, he lashed out.

His physical reactions always appeared to be unprovoked and I knew some of the other boys would goad him on since he was easily manipulated. But in the end he was the one hurting the other kids in spite of whatever they were doing to get him into trouble. I lived under the daily stress of not only getting a bad report, but also of the school telling me it was the last straw, that Henry could no longer be a student there and then what would I do? I had a full-time job and finding a new preschool in an area where there was a year's waiting list for most places was nearly impossible. Fortunately for us, Henry's preschool was able to deal with his behavior, calling in a specialist from the public school they worked with to come in and observe him in the classroom and make suggestions for how to better deal with and, ultimately, prevent his outbursts.

My son's diagnosis wasn't exactly a shock as I had suspected since he was a baby that he was showing signs of autism. His hyper-focus on what he was working on, the inability to carry on a two-sided conversation, his not seeing the world from any perspective other than his own and various sensory issues were early clues. On one hand, it was good to have a diagnosis to some degree, but on the other it was daunting to know that he faced a lifetime of struggle in understanding others and having to learn things that come naturally to most people.

Specialists refer to Asperger's as high-functioning autism but it is still disabling when you lack social skills and the ability to moderate your emotions. And then there are all the so-called "comorbid" issues that tend to accompany the diagnosis: anxiety disorder, sensory processing disorder, obsessive-compulsive disorder (OCD) and attention deficit hyperactivity disorder (ADHD). These are the daily issues that made life difficult for him and, in turn, the rest of our family. His behavior and comfort level over the next few years became increasingly disruptive and this, combined with his inability to manage his anxiety and OCD, had us turning to medication for help.

I'd be lying if I said that I never thought that somehow it was my fault that my son had autism. Was it something that happened during my pregnancy? Was I too anxious and it elevated my cortisol levels and made him more susceptible to this? I had avoided the more commonly known toxin issue at the time (phthalates and nail polish), but those toxins affected reproductive organs and not brain development. Were all those Rh-immune globulin shots I received during my pregnancy, used to prevent Rh incompatibility and chock-full of mercury, part of the cause? Or was a genetic predisposition to being on the autistic range triggered by some environmental factor the reason for his neurological problems?

We have a history of autistic-like behaviors in my side of the family—tic disorders, anxiety issues, lack of social skills, they run the gamut. But why was Henry more severely affected than the rest of us? Was he at a distinct disadvantage by being born at a time when we are all bearing a fairly heavy body burden of toxins?

The bones of an 85-year-old

"I just want to prepare you that one of the tests we are looking at is for cancer." These words shocked me out of my diatribe about what the cause of my husband's back pain might be. I had just spent the last few minutes on my cell phone while driving to the hospital where Hank had just been admitted, explaining to our doctor what I thought was the reason why my 38-year-old husband wasn't able to walk. Why he was in such unbearable pain.

In retrospect, it was wishful thinking that something simple like piriformis syndrome (tight muscles in the legs that can pull on your lower back) would be the reason for Hank's slow decline over the past several months. The lab work ultimately indicated there was something much more serious going on. I would fully come to realize and accept in the week that followed, as he came close to death in the ICU of Swedish Hospital, that cancer was eating my husband and partner of 18 years from the inside of his bones.

Unlike Henry's diagnosis, my husband's diagnosis was an absolute, breathtaking shock. His physical problems had started months earlier when he noticed his running times were slowing. Here was a man who exercised religiously and, frankly, was the healthiest person I had ever met, but I just figured he was getting older. And it was hard to commiserate with his "slow" run times of 9 minutes per mile when, even at my fittest, I rarely saw the underbelly of 10. Over the ensuing months, he started developing back pain. Again, I chalked it up to old age. My family has chronic back pain issues so it just seemed like he was finally catching up. It wasn't until his back pain started becoming more debilitating and he could barely walk that an MRI was ordered. But nothing looked out of the ordinary.

When Hank was referred to a rheumatologist and full lab tests were ordered we were alarmed, but by then we just wanted to find out what the problem was. Unfortunately, before we even got any answers, my husband's back pain became so bad that, one morning before work, he couldn't move and I took him to the emergency room. Actually, I had to call a medical transport to take him to the hospital because the slightest movement caused excruciating pain. He later told me it was a good thing I wasn't in the room when they moved him because the pain was so intense. I didn't tell him that I was waiting in the living room with my fingers plugging my ears because I couldn't bear to hear him screaming.

In the ER they couldn't resolve his pain regardless of the amount of narcotics he was given and they admitted him to the hospital. After a number of tests, the definitive one involving a bone marrow biopsy, Hank was diagnosed with multiple myeloma, a cancer of the plasma cells in the bone marrow. It is extremely uncommon in 38-year-old men and, by the time Hank was diagnosed, his disease was so advanced that 94% of his bone marrow plasma cells were cancerous and his bones were as brittle as an 85-year-old's.

To fast-forward through all the gruesome cancer treatments, after a month in the hospital, followed by aggressive chemotherapy, tandem stem cell transplants and more hospital stays, three years later Hank was doing well. He was back on chemotherapy but able to work full-time and, most importantly, he had beaten the three-year death sentence they initially gave him. Based on the staging of his disease and the type of cancer, the average lifespan of a patient in his situation, with treatment, is three years.

The question that kept me up at night was why would an otherwise completely healthy young individual be stricken with an uncommon form of cancer generally only seen in people over the age of 65? More alarmingly, the incidence of this cancer was trending downward, age-wise, and doctors were diagnosing more and more young men with this disease. And it was being seen more particularly in firefighters as well as those who helped in the World Trade Center cleanup. Exposure to environmental toxins has been suspected in both cases. Again, I'd be lying if I said I hadn't racked my brains trying to figure out what genetic factors coupled with environmental exposure could have led to such a horrible outcome. I had (and still have) my suspicions, but we'll never know for sure.

Trying to make sense of it all

Armed with this history of family disease and troubled by the increased rates of both conditions, I was further appalled at what I was reading as I was going through *Slow Death by Rubber Duck*. The authors of the book had set up an experiment to see if they could increase the levels of toxins in their bodies, otherwise known as their toxin body burden, by locking themselves away for a few days and using common products and eating commonplace foods. These products were high in toxins such as phthalates (a plasticizer common in PVC and other materials) and parabens (used as preservatives) as well as foods that were high in mercury and packaged in bisphenol-A (BPA) or cooked in Teflon. The laundry list of chemicals and their associated health implications were truly frightening and I wondered how much I had been affected by this same chemical soup.

I was intrigued by the blood and urine tests they underwent to see the before and after effects of their experiment and started thinking about not just what kind of impact these toxins had on me but also, if the authors of this book could increase their body burden so dramatically in a few days, what kind of measurable reduction could be made over a few months' time with a dramatic decrease in exposure to these chemicals? And that is how this book and project were born.

The Non-Toxic Avenger

The mission to lower my own personal body burden of toxins began with my getting tested for a wide array of toxins, both those under my control by my own product usage and exposure and those that are considered background exposure (that is, those toxins that exist in the environment [air, water and soil] and that I have little control over). Once the initial testing was complete, I systematically removed every single possible toxin source from my environment that I could reasonably remove, engaged in a "detox" under the care of a doctor and, at the end, got retested to see what, if any, impact I had made on my original body burden levels.

> *We absorb so many synthetic chemicals during an average lifetime that, according to some reports, when we die our bodies decompose more slowly today than if we had died just three decades ago.*
>
> Randall Fitzgerald,
> *The Hundred-Year Lie*

Going into this project I was fully aware that I might not test high in some toxins given my aversion to chemicals. However, I could have been stuffed with more toxins than I thought. I was also aware that there were some toxins I had less control over (in regards to exposure) and that those that are stored in body fat are harder to remove than others. That's where the detox at the end of the project came into play.

Lab testing

When I initially started thinking of doing this project, I researched which labs other authors and toxicologists were using for body burden testing and contacted them directly to see how to order the tests. It turned out to be much more onerous than I expected.

Through a personal contact (Dr. Steven Gilbert, a friend of my brother and who just happens to be a toxicologist), I was connected with Erika Schreder, a staff scientist at Washington Toxics Coalition who led the Toxic-Free Legacy Coalition's Pollution in People study[1] and was a participant in the Environmental Working Group's Human Toxome Project.

Since the Toxic-Free Legacy Coalition had done a series of body burden testing on Washington State residents and most of the tests were similar to the ones I was interested in getting done, Erika was a great resource. One issue that she brought up in conversation was the quality of testing and detection levels depending on the lab used. It wasn't something that I would have thought of initially, so going with well-regarded laboratories for analysis would be key in trusting the results of my lab tests.

Another issue Erika mentioned was regarding the difficulty of a single individual, rather than a research institution or a medical facility, gaining access to some of these laboratories and their tests. Apparently, other journalists who were trying to get body burden testing had been refused by one of the larger labs. So, getting access to certain tests could potentially prove to be a problem. After our conversation, I was initially resigned to not getting all the tests done that I wanted.

I'll go into much more detail about the toxins I was targeting in short order, but just to introduce them, the ones I was interested in getting tested for were: phthalates, parabens, polybrominated diphenyl ether flame retardants (PBDEs), heavy metals (mercury, lead, arsenic), perfluorinated compounds (nonstick chemicals), pesticides, persistent toxic chemicals (like dichlorodiphenyltrichloroethane [DDT] and polychlorinated biphenyls [PCBs]), bisphenol A (BPA) and triclosan (an antibacterial).

One of the major laboratories I ended up using was Metametrix Clinical Labs, which offered a series of Environmental Toxicities Lab Panels (the panels are really just a grouping of similar toxins all done at the same time). More importantly, the lab panel information and patient information were easily accessible on their website. After contacting Metametrix, I was informed that I would need to work with a local healthcare provider in Seattle to arrange the blood draws and the provider would send the samples to the lab. From the list of providers they sent, I chose a doctor from Bastyr University, a well-regarded alternative medical school and clinic in Seattle.

Deciding on the tests

Ready with the list of Metametrix tests I was interested in undergoing, I met with Dr. John Hibbs, a specialist in environmental medicine and an expert in detoxification at Bastyr. I initially thought that he would merely be arranging the specific panels offered by Metametrix, but he was interested in helping me find the labs and tests for all the toxins I was interested in testing, not just the ones offered by Metametrix.

We discussed alternative methods of toxicity testing that blood, urine and hair tests couldn't detect since several of the toxins that I wanted to test for are stored in body fat and don't show up as easily in the more basic tests. Dr. Hibbs mentioned some toxicity testing research that had been done using fat biopsies, which generally aren't done because they are invasive and expensive and leave scarring. But if I wanted to really know what the levels of insecticides (like DDT) and heavy metals (like mercury) were, fat biopsy testing would be far more definitive than blood and urine testing.

Dr. Hibbs and I also talked about therapies for detoxification that I could undergo as I moved further into the project. No decision was made about what exactly I would do, but I was given some handouts describing diet, exercise, supplements and sweat therapy that I could undertake to assist in ridding my body of the toxins that get stored in body fat and other tissues. All of this seemed reasonable until I got home and read the detox regimen in detail. I was in for a few surprises.

At this initial meeting we left it that his team would research which tests they could arrange and how much they would cost, including options for fat biopsies. Based on that information, I would choose the final test selection. Since full body burden testing can cost upward of $10,000, I wanted to make sure that I didn't go too crazy with selecting too many tests because I would be doing follow-up testing later. And I wanted to stay on an expenses budget of less than $5,000 during the project.

As if disfiguring fat biopsies weren't enough, right after this meeting I had an email conversation with a good friend of mine who publicly goes by the name Greenpa and writes the blog *Little Blog in the Big Woods*. He's been living off the grid for more than

30 years, and has all but a hair's breadth of a PhD in biology. He was suggesting that another definitive test would be breast milk testing since fat-soluble toxins are excreted in breast milk. Since I was no longer lactating (my kids being seven and eight at the time), but knowing that I'm game for pretty much anything, he suggested that I try prolactin therapy to reinstate lactation to rid myself of toxins as well as do some testing.

The approach sounded more like a study in lactation and how many toxins show up in the fore versus hind milk (basically, the fore milk is high in carbs and the hind milk is high in lipids, aka fats). In any case, in spite of its potential relevance and my own curiosity about how many toxins I was feeding my children as babies, I wasn't interested in pumping myself with hormones to test that theory. I figured it was best to leave it to the researchers and women who are lactating naturally to solve that puzzle.

Not getting ahead of myself

One of the problems with doing the research for this book and not getting started with the actual testing and project right away was the fact that it was nearly impossible to read all the data on the potential health consequences of the toxins and not want to stop using these chemicals immediately. My initial reaction was to go through all my cabinets and closets and toss out everything containing any of the chemicals I was focusing on. The research was that scary. But I also didn't want to skew the lab tests by going into them already precleaned. That would defeat the purpose of the two sets of tests.

Since I was already using a number of nasty chemicals, in spite of the "naturalness" trumpeted on the packaging, I resolved to continue using them until I got my body burden tested. On one hand it was kind of a relief to throw caution to the wind and continue using and consuming products that I knew were potentially harmful to me all in the name of "research." It felt somewhat decadent to drink Diet Coke in a plastic bottle. But on the other hand, I knew some products had enough potential health consequences that I couldn't wait to stop using them.

I must admit that, even before I got this project in gear, I tossed almost all of my kids' bathroom products (except toothpaste) that contained suspicious chemicals and replaced them with completely non-toxic ones. And my husband was banned from using anything even remotely toxic or carcinogenic. Since he already had cancer, he didn't need any more exposure from additional toxins. I especially worried about some of the skin and hair care products he was using and I got those out of the house as soon as I could find a replacement.

I felt comfortable going ahead and removing the toxins my family was exposed to while continuing to use these products myself. I wanted to maintain, in a sense, a "real-life" exposure and to have test results representative of someone who mostly chooses low-risk, natural or organic products. In the meantime, it drove me a tad crazy because I saw all these toxic products around me that I wanted to get rid of, but couldn't just yet.

One more thing

Before getting too far along in this, I should mention my own health problems that may have been affected by environmental toxins. At the time of starting this project, I was a fairly healthy 40-year-old and generally didn't have any complaints except for the occasional migraine. My skin burned relatively easily and I had a high propensity for getting freckles and moles. I used to always joke that I'd be the first person between my husband and me to have health issues, either from skin cancer or a stroke (since individuals who have the kind of migraines I have—that is, with aura—are at a much higher risk of having a stroke). The fact that I was still going strong, relatively speaking, wasn't what I expected. I expected I would be the one with the health problems and my husband would be the healthy one. So far, though, I was wrong.

However, about two weeks before I first met with Dr. Hibbs, I began experiencing some unusual symptoms that hadn't really abated by our meeting. Pretty much overnight, I started having numbness, tingling and, sometimes, burning in my hands, arms, legs and feet. This is generally called peripheral neuropathy and the only reason I know this is because peripheral neuropathy is one of the side-effects of the chemo drugs and immune suppressants my husband is on. It wasn't particularly painful, but it was annoying and, in my case, unnerving (pardon the pun) since I didn't know what was causing it.

Add to that the fact that I am highly prone to being a hypochondriac. Since my husband was diagnosed with cancer I've gotten a little better about it, but over the years I have convinced myself on numerous occasions that I had some major health problem or other. The simplest thing always escalated, in my mind, to brain cancer or imminent death. For example, a few months after my son was born and I was on maternity leave, I was absolutely convinced I was going blind. If I looked at the rug just so, I couldn't see what I thought was a large section in my visual field.

I tend to be more sensitive about my vision strictly because, right before I get a migraine, I get what's called visual aura. It's hard to describe, but basically it's like you are looking through a kaleidoscope. Everything is jumbled up and colors are swirling around; you can't see faces and you can't read and, generally, I find it to be more annoying than the migraine pain itself. So I have always hyper-focused on what my vision is doing since it's the first sign I'm getting a migraine. Or having a stroke or developing a brain tumor, of course.

Back then, I spent a whole week testing my vision as I sat there during those many hours of nursing sessions, putting my hand up to my eyes, testing what I could and couldn't see. I was all but convinced I had some sort of brain tumor pushing on my optical nerve and causing my blindness. I finally decided to look it up online. Well, it turned out I was just hyper-focusing on my blind spots. Everyone has them—they're where the optic nerve goes into the back of your eye and, for a small spot in your field of vision, you can't see. Some people are able to see them more than others and, I suspect, if you spend days practicing like I was, you get pretty good at it. I think when I finally told my husband what was going on he thought I was off my rocker. But then again, he's also a hypochondriac. Not a good trait to have when you have cancer.

Anyway, this particular time with the numbness and tingling was no different. I tried to stuff down my fears of the ever-looming brain tumor and decided that maybe something like multiple sclerosis was a better choice this time around. The symptoms were certainly more appropriate. Or how about something rheumatic? Unfortunately, the symptoms didn't match and I wasn't really fatigued, so that ruled out a host of other scary things. I initially figured it was from a pinched nerve or something since I had been doing a lot of outdoor work involving heavy lifting the few days prior, but the fact that I was experiencing the symptoms in all of my extremities pointed to something else.

A metabolic problem was what my family doctor initially suspected when I went in to see her after experiencing the symptoms for over a week. She did a basic neurological exam and ran blood tests, suspecting that I was B12 deficient, which causes the same symptoms. But all my blood work came back normal—iron, thyroid, blood count—everything was fine. My Vitamin D was very low and my B12 was in the low-normal range, so I started taking supplements.

The extra B12 seemed to help, or so I thought, but then the symptoms came back. In fact, they were intermittent. Some days I didn't notice any symptoms and other days they were really distracting. I finally made the connection one morning when I was about to apply some sunscreen. It was a new one that I had just started using. In fact, I had just started using it around the same time my symptoms started. Not wanting to jump on some new crackpot theory about the origins of my problems, since I was previously convinced it was the B12 issue, I decided to stop using this sunscreen and see if the neuropathy went away.

Thinking back, the worst episodes were right after I had used a lot of sunscreen, either because I was working outside in the yard (the weekend before all this started) or after we had gone to an outdoor pool, when I really slathered it on. The following day would bring the worst symptoms I had. And since I didn't use that particular sunscreen every day, due to our cloudy summers in Seattle, that might explain why some days I didn't have any symptoms and other days I did.

At this point, it was just a theory, but I decided to do some research on chemical reactions, nerve issues and sunscreen ingredients. I didn't find anything definitive linking the two, but I did find some information on multiple chemical sensitivities and symptoms. A lot of the symptoms that I have are always attributed to low blood sugar, and migraines mimic the symptoms of multiple chemical sensitivities. I never really made any connection between the two and, since there are so many possible contributing factors that cause these symptoms, it could have just been absolute coincidence. But, that said, I am very sensitive to fragrances and will get migraines if exposed to overly scented products.

During medical consultations, the concept that chemical exposure may have contributed in some way to a patient's problem doesn't even enter the doctor's head.

Physician and toxins
expert Paula Baillie-Hamilton,
The Hundred-Year Lie

As another example, the week my numbness and tingling symptoms first started my brother-in-law came to visit for his high school reunion. He brought with him his arsenal of scented body products. He prides himself on smelling good and has quite the display of colognes in his home bathroom. His shower at home is also fully stocked with drugstore scented shampoos and body washes and the like, which, to me, are very sickly and sweet-smelling. I find them very irritating. The day he arrived, I could smell his soaps and whatnot wafting upstairs from the basement bathroom he was using. Between that and his cologne, and probably other factors, I got a migraine. Fortunately it was short-lived, but I couldn't help thinking, when I was lying in bed with my eyes closed, watching the kaleidoscope swirls, that the trigger must have been all that fragrance.

Looking back, my fragrance theory makes sense but, since I'm of the mind to want to have more proof than mere coincidence and conjecture, I wanted to really see if I did have chemical sensitivities, particularly in relation to the sunscreen I was using. So I stopped using the sunscreen and waited to see if I continued experiencing the symptoms. If they didn't go away, the next step was to get an MRI of my head. Which, as my dad was joking, would most likely turn up nothing. Or so I hoped.

Where did the bad stuff go?

As I was waiting to schedule the body burden tests, I began working on other parts of the project which included identifying some of the easier things to eliminate. But that raised the question of what I would do with all the stuff I deemed to be toxic. Should I throw it out, flush it, dump it down the drain, recycle it or donate it?

If a product (like a body lotion) was partially used and I could salvage the packaging for recycling, I would go ahead and recycle it. I didn't want to pour chemical products down the drain and unleash it on the waterways to cause mutant fish, algal blooms or worse. I suspected each product would require an independent decision on how I would dispose of it.

As for clothing, jewelry or other consumer goods that were still usable, I planned on donating them to local donation centers like Value Village, Goodwill or the Salvation Army. I hated thinking that my once coveted items were being donated at the potential health expense of someone else, but it wasn't like I was donating nuclear waste to unwitting consumers.

The argument for donating potentially hazardous products (that didn't qualify for hazardous waste disposal) was the same for getting rid of environmentally unfriendly products. Some environmentalists recommend getting rid of partially used products for free on Craigslist or Freecycle, but I think sharing personal care products is potentially a hazard in itself. Others feel that by donating the product you are passing the problem onto someone else. However, I'd argue that the individual buying or taking the donated product would have purchased something similar anyway, and in the end, you are removing it from the waste stream and reducing the demand.

While I wanted to prevent throwing out as much as possible, I also needed to get rid of a number of items from pretty much every avenue of my life and the bulk of them would be donated or sold on Craigslist. I could see the ad: "Potentially hazardous contaminated children's plastic toys. Mint. Retail $25. Yours for only $5. Lead poisoning included."

Lab test snafus

As I initially suspected, I had a tough time gaining access to one of the labs that does the BPA, triclosan, flame retardants and a couple of the other toxin tests I was interested in getting. Since I was working with physicians to get the testing done, this lab assumed that I was doing the tests for medical diagnostic purposes rather than for research. They claimed they were unable to do any testing for medical purposes because they were not CLIA (that is, Clinical Laboratory Improvement Amendments) certified. This certification is a U.S. Department of Health and Human Services regulation over clinical laboratories.[2]

Bastyr could have pursued setting up something with this lab, but since I was the only patient doing the test for nonmedical purposes, it wouldn't really be worth their time. And furthermore, there was still the issue of the lab not running tests for a single individual. From conversations I had with other people, I had the impression that setting up the test at the lab is expensive for only one sample. For a group of people getting tested (as for a research program with multiple samples) it made sense, but not for an individual.

Because of this, I ended up narrowing down the list of toxin tests that I would get done and started working out the pricing. Fortunately it ended up being a lot cheaper than I had originally thought. As mentioned before, a full body burden testing can cost upward of $10,000. Since I was not getting tested for the full range of toxins and was focusing only on specific ones, the costs were less. In addition, during this last go-round on tests, we decided that blood and 24-hour urine samples were sufficient for the heavy metal toxicity testing and so we skipped the hair tests.

My budget for the first set of tests was $2,500 and, because I was restricted from getting tested for at least four types of toxins, I ended up coming in way below that. The good news was that this freed my budget up to spend money on others things in the project itself rather than spending all of my budgeted money on testing.

What's so bad about a little lead?

By now, one might wonder what all the fuss is with the chemicals I had targeted in the testing as well as the other ones I was determined to avoid during the project, even if I wasn't getting tested for them. Most of them are carcinogenic (meaning they can cause cancer), disrupt hormones in some fashion or cause long-term health issues like diabetes, heart disease or worse. There are thousands of different chemicals in the products most of us use daily and there are few standards for testing their safety.

Chemicals like BPA can cause abnormal development of the brain, behavioral changes and a predisposition to cancer, diabetes and heart disease. Teflon and other nonstick-type chemicals (these include water- and stain-resistant coatings and the linings of a lot of food packaging like chip bags and candy bar wrappers) are likely human carcinogens. These nonstick toxins (generally referred to as PFC or PFOA, which I'll go into later) are associated with low sperm counts — which isn't an issue for me — and animal studies have shown they can alter the development of mammary tissue — which does concern me, outside of the cancer risk.

Flame retardants, which are in more consumer products and clothing than one can imagine, are linked to cancer, thyroid hormone disruption and a lower IQ. Formaldehyde, which is just as pervasive, can cause respiratory cancer, leukemia and asthma. Lead can cause brain, kidney and heart damage in kids and adults, lower a child's IQ and shorten his or her attention span, and increase hyperactivity and aggressive behavior. Some of those issues we already have in our household.

Phthalates (found in fragrances and plastics) lower testosterone levels, which is a problem in both males and females. Exposure during development has been linked to malformations of the male reproductive tract (that nail polish issue again) as well as testicular cancer. It can also contribute to obesity, reduced fertility and behavior changes.

While PCBs and DDT were banned decades ago, they persist in the environment and show up in our bodies via the food we eat. Kids with greater exposure to PCBs have lower birth weights and slower growth including brain development. It's considered a human carcinogen as well. DDT, another carcinogen, is harmful to the nervous system, potentially causing lasting neurological and cognitive problems. Since it's also an estrogen mimic (it acts like estrogen in the body), it can cause hormone disruption.

These are just a few of the chemicals I focused on while going through five months of lifestyle avoidance where I eliminated or limited our exposure to these toxins. Since most of them were linked to cancer, neurological problems, hormonal disruption and behavioral issues, they were also more of a concern for my family than the average family. I hoped that by eliminating them we would see a reduction in symptoms: behavioral improvements for my son and cancer reduction for my husband. With less of a toxic load triggering these issues, I hoped that our bodies would recover faster and our immune systems would be better primed to deal with the underlying problems we already had rather than trying to fight off something new. It was a long shot, but a worthy effort I wanted to undertake nonetheless.

Getting Started

Clean air

One thing I didn't have a tremendous amount of control over during this project was outdoor air quality. I'll be addressing indoor air and toxins later in the book, but unless I was planning on wearing a respirator outside for five months, the best I could do was to try not to go outside on poor air quality days. Since we were heading into late summer when I began this project and the weather had been really mild, even for Seattle, our air quality had been good. That's what all that rain we experienced was good for. We generally have some burn ban days in the fall so I was determined to pay a little closer attention to when the air was nasty.

If the outdoor air quality was bad, I tried to stay inside where I had more control over what I was breathing in. Because I was taking a leave of absence from work to write this book, my only really necessary trips during the day were walking down to school to drop off and pick up the kids. Otherwise, I could hunker down inside if necessary.

Speaking of school, right before classes started we took a short trip over Labor Day weekend to a cabin in Mt. Rainier National Park. It's a beautiful area and we went for some hikes up on the mountain. As we were resting, having a snack and enjoying breathtaking views of the glaciers, I was imploring the kids to take deep breaths of fresh mountain air, explaining that it was probably the cleanest air they would ever breathe in. Unfortunately, that fresh mountain air wasn't exactly as clean as I thought it was.

A few days after we came back from our trip, I received an e-mail regarding an article about airborne pollutants in our national parks.[1] Right on the accompanying webpage was a picture featuring Mt. Rainier. Eight years ago the National Parks Service started a study of airborne contaminants in western national parks, focusing on a number of parks including Glacier, Olympic, Mt. Rainier, Denali and Gates of the Arctic.

What they found was that, of the 100 or more toxic substances tested for, 70 were found, including some chemicals that had been banned for decades. Many fish in these parks had reached or exceeded the threshold of contaminants — including mercury and DDT and other pesticides — that made them unsafe for consumption by humans and other animals that eat them. If alpine fish were that contaminated, what did it mean for lake fish and other aquatic species at lower altitudes, presumably closer to the source? It sounded like I would be crossing off fish from my diet during this project since it seemed that there were no fish in the food chain that hadn't been affected by toxins.

The researchers also found, understandably, that many of the contaminants in the parks were specific to the geographic area where they were located and what businesses and industries were in the area. In other words, some pollutants like flame retardants and pesticides were in higher concentrations if industry or agriculture using those contaminants were nearby.

In any case, the air in Mt. Rainier National Park was definitely cleaner than the air in the city, so I don't regret all the deep breathing I subjected my family to, but our days of pristine air and water in remote areas are long gone. Fortunately, studies like these can help change policies. Because of the research and findings in our national parks, the Environmental Protection Agency (EPA) has already banned some pesticides. And who knows, maybe in 30 years my children will be able to take their own kids to the national parks and the air and water will be cleaner than they are today.

Sparkles, jewels and dangly items

I spent a day in early September going over what jewelry I commonly wear and whether or not there might be a problem with heavy metal toxicity. Until each piece was tested I wouldn't know for sure but, with the scares of lead in jewelry made in China, and now cadmium, which has been known to hinder brain development in young children and cause kidney damage if ingested, if I didn't know where it was made and what it was made out of, I considered that piece questionable and stopped wearing it. And this included quite a few pieces that weren't pure metal or stainless steel. It's not like I was mouthing my jewelry, but it was in direct contact with my skin for a huge chunk of the day, so it was possible it was somehow contributing to my heavy metal load.

I had a lot of earrings which were probably just stainless steel, but several of them were of unknown origin and materials. Those went in the donation bin. I didn't have any questionable earrings that had any sentimental value and I didn't feel like I had to hold onto them. As for the rest of my head, I have my nose pierced, but all my jewelry was stainless steel, so no problems there. Moving down, I had a lot of necklaces. Most of them were chains with metal of known origin but I also had some cheap jewelry and I wasn't sure what it was made out of. I suspected those pieces probably contained some lead with a sprinkling of cadmium. I saved a few of them to analyze at the end of the project.

A decent x-ray fluorescence (XRF) analyzer gun can distinguish between lead on the surface of an object and lead in the substrate (what it's made out of). It is extremely useful for screening consumer products like toys and will test for not just lead but also other toxins like cadmium, mercury and arsenic.[2] In addition to toy screening, an XRF analyzer can be used to test fashion jewelry, furniture and apparel for lead. My plan was to bring a pile of toys, jewelry, dishes and other things in for testing at the end of the project. I just needed to find someone with an analyzer gun who was willing to humor me.

My wedding ring and engagement ring, the latter of which I don't wear very often, weren't an issue. I didn't wear any metal bracelets but I was wearing a braided friendship bracelet that my daughter, Emma, and I both have identical versions of. She picked them out on Mother's Day the previous year at one of our local farmers' markets. I honestly don't know what kind of material it's made out of—I think it's some sort of cotton/poly blend. It wasn't exactly my color style (it's very Rastafarian), but Emma picked it out, so I ran with it. Anyway, the fibers were brightly colored so I don't know what kind of potential toxins were used in the pigment. And furthermore, I didn't know how many remained, potentially leaching out when wet, and what kind of issue this could pose. Perhaps it would be something else to set aside for testing with the XRF gun. In the meantime, it had too much sentimental value and I kept it on.

Seeing double

I had three pairs of glasses at the start of this project, two of which had frames made from some sort of plastic. I had one pair that I rarely wore that was made of titanium steel, but the nose pieces were made out of those little plastic pieces and the metal around the earpiece had a plastic covering. Most nose pads are made of silicone or acetate, but they also can be made of polyvinyl chloride (PVC). I'm not sure which material mine was made from.

All the lenses in my glasses were polycarbonate with a hard plastic coating. The polycarbonate material in eyeglass (and sunglass) lenses is produced by the reaction of BPA and phosgene, a toxic, colorless gas that gained infamy as a chemical weapon during World War I. Of course, since some of the original materials and, furthermore, the lenses didn't make direct contact with my skin, I wasn't going to worry about it. If the polycarbonate material did rest on my skin there was the potential of the BPA leaching onto my skin from heat and sweat, although the probability would be very low.[3] BPA is a potential endocrine disruptor. In animal studies, it has appeared to be released from polycarbonate animal cages into water at room temperature and it may have been responsible for enlargement of the reproductive organs of female mice. Here the risk was small and I didn't expect any enlarged reproductive organs from my lenses.

But I was still wondering about those frames. The safer pair of glasses was probably going to be the titanium ones, but the prescription in that pair was the oldest. I didn't have any all-metal glasses to work with and, I suspected, contacts have got to be far worse as far as materials go. I wasn't sure if it was possible to even get actual glass lenses anymore, but I was comfortable enough with the low risk of polycarbonate or other plastics. I didn't like that the toxins went into making them, but from the consumption point of view, the toxicity to me personally (although still indirectly through its manufacture) was, for now, undetectable. It was possible to get new nose pads made from natural rubber[4] or glass,[5] but the risk wasn't high enough to warrant the effort.

I was running into the same issues with my sunglasses in that they were made from plastic and had a nose pad of unidentifiable origin. Sunglasses are not optional for me since sunlight triggers migraines, but because I live in Seattle and this project was occurring during the "low-light" months, my exposure would be somewhat less. Unless I was able to find some inexpensive natural-framed sunglasses, I decided to punt on them or, at the very least, get some glass nose pads.

PVC-free dreams

At the beginning of the school year, or really, a month or two before school started, the Environmental Working Group and other nonprofits were sending out emails to environmental bloggers about choosing non-toxic school supplies for the new school year. The lists were fairly comprehensive and I was delighted to see commonly found manufacturers such as Avery, PaperMate and

Faber-Castell on the list, rather than some difficult to find, special order brands. I fully planned on using the guide to equip my two children with school supplies for the year.

After downloading one of the lists, I forwarded an email to the parents of the kids in my children's classes recommending that they take a look at the Center for Health, Environment & Justice's PVC-free School Supplies list, which also explained the dangers of PVC in the classroom environment.[6] The general problem with PVC is that it is unique among plastics because it contains chemical additives such as phthalates, lead and cadmium which can be toxic to a child's health. An even bigger problem with PVC, however, is that these chemical additives can leach out or evaporate into the air over time, posing unnecessary dangers to children. And because children are at risk from even low concentration exposures to these toxic chemicals it's important to not have a ton of PVC school supplies off-gassing in the classroom.

That email elicited a few responses of thanks back from the parents and word that they were forwarding it to other parents. I felt that the more parents who paid attention to what they were buying for school, the less overall exposure to PVC the kids in the class would endure during the school day. It was with good intentions that I planned on making sure that all the supplies we provided were non-toxic, particularly with writing this book, since I wanted to set a good example.

However, two things stood in my way and prevented me from doing so. First, Seattle Public Schools (SPS) notoriously waits until the last minute to send out school supply lists. A few years back, they used to send out preliminary lists for different grade levels earlier in August. We would dutifully buy our school supplies only to later receive a completely different list from the actual teacher of the classroom the kids were assigned to. It was frustrating to say the least. SPS no longer sends out the preliminary supplies list, and now waits until the classroom assignments have been made and the teachers' lists have been compiled, mailing all the paperwork out together.

The biggest problem with this process is that you don't receive the school supplies list until a few days before school starts and the supplies are due. This particular year we received the list on the Friday before Labor Day as we were leaving for our trip down to the refreshing air of Mt. Rainier. Since we were gone all weekend, we would only have one day to buy all the necessary school supplies. So, if there was anything on the list that was difficult to find as a PVC-free version, it would either have to wait or I'd have to scramble and try to find it. But I knew this already and I planned to do what I could.

Unfortunately, the larger issue was really not working with my mom. My mom is a woman who loves a good sale. And, as a retiree, she has a lot of time on her hands to work on it. She had been talking all summer about making sure she got the school supply lists because she had been watching the sales at places like Office Depot and other stores that carry school supplies. In general, she has no problems with making multiple trips out to the store just to take advantage of the loss-leaders for the week and had been excited about getting this and that supply for mere pennies.

While we were up on Mt. Rainier, feeding deer and hiking among wildflowers, my mom took it upon herself to do some house-sitting. She stops by frequently for a variety of reasons, but on this occasion she saw the school supply lists that I had left out on the counter as a reminder to myself to get cracking on them as soon as we got home from our trip. However, while we were gone she beavered away on the task, going out and buying everything on the lists and neatly leaving us two paper bags — one for Emma, with all her supplies, and one for Henry, with all his.

On one hand, I was quite relieved and appreciative that she had gone through the trouble of taking care of one of my least favorite chores; on the other hand, I was disappointed that I didn't get a chance to buy the PVC-free school supplies I had promised myself I would do. I couldn't blame her. I didn't tell her about my PVC-free dreams, and I knew she would pretty much go to town with the lists if she saw them. The good thing, really, was that none of the items on the lists were inherently made from PVC. There were no binders or the like on the list, just paper, pencils, folders, few things that, generally, are made with PVC. I can't say I looked too closely, though. We were in a mad rush to get everything else ready for school, so I didn't go sniffing through the bags. I figured ignorance was bliss.

The first week of school, one of the moms from my daughter's class came over to me asking about this book and thanking me for the email I sent out. It took me a few seconds to remember what she was talking about since it had been a month and a half and I am generally always sending out some strange email or other and losing track of them. She had taken the PVC-free supply list and used it to buy all of her school supplies from it. At least someone had managed to do it!

One thing I did have control over was replacing Henry's PVC-laden backpacks. I didn't feel too bad about getting rid of them. They were in sorry shape, being poorly made and shredding to pieces over the years. One had just blown out the bottom at the end of the last school year, and the other, older back-up one was missing half of its plastic PVC decorations. I managed to find a new one at Land's End that I believed would last him more than one year and, furthermore, was PVC free. While I was making the order for the new backpack, I also got two lunchboxes that were PVC and lead free. Most fancy lunch bags are made with PVC and many of them, if they keep food cold, contain lead. I didn't want the kids' food stewing in a PVC 'n' lead mix all day long.

What's that on your lunch tray?

It was during the second week of school, just after the school bell rang, that the principal came on the loudspeaker to make a few announcements, ending with, "Today for lunch you have the choice of a hamburger, cheeseburger or cheese quesadilla. Mmm, mmm good." According to another parent, my friend Ron, this lunch announcement script went on every day and always ended with the "Mmm, mmm good" part. Ron and I both lamented this sales pitch because, honestly, our school lunches were kind of disgusting and this description gave a false sense of not only nutrition but good taste.

I know the school district meant well and they tried to meet some standards of nutrition, but for the most part the food was sketchy. At least from my observation. The couple of times I had gone into the lunchroom to meet up with my kids, I always left with a sad, sick feeling in my stomach after watching the children who bought their lunch eat this microwave-heated, encased-in-plastic meal.

Unfortunately, our school did not have a kitchen that was geared for actually cooking food, prepping food or much else. I didn't get the impression that there was much difference in any of the other schools in the district because they all shared the same menu. I figured that somewhere, someone was prepping the food, packaging it and transporting it out to the schools. And then you only needed one person (Miss Molly in our case) to reheat the food at the school and distribute it to the hungry masses.

My main concern with the food offered—not that my children ate it, though—was the plastic components and how they were heated with the plastic cellophane wrapper still on it. Another issue was the milk: where it came from and what hormones, if any, the cows were subjected to. It turned out, according to the district website, that all the milk on offer was rBST (an artificial growth hormone) free. But it was not organic and I assumed that the cows were fed grain and a healthy dollop of antibiotics to counteract the health implications of milk cows eating grain, which is not something they evolved to do. The underlying issue was that the antibiotics fed to the milk herd could potentially get passed on through the milk to the child.

Unneeded antibiotics aren't good for any human, but they are particularly unneeded in young, growing bodies where the health effects are not quite known. Are antibiotics a toxin? Not per se, but any chemical not inherently part of the nature of the food certainly wasn't something I wanted in my children's bodies. Sometimes (rarely) my kids liked buying the school milk and would charge it up without my knowing about it until I got the bill. My feeling was, if they wanted milk at lunch, they could bring it from home and I could manage the toxic input of their food choices.

Lice!

A few weeks into the school year we got sent home a note from my son's third grade classroom notifying us that "one or more cases of head lice have been found or reported in your child's classroom." I used to completely freak out when we started receiving these dreaded letters in his kindergarten class and mentally pledged to shave everyone bald, but I got used to the letters over the years and so far, knock on wood, neither of my children has gotten lice from school or elsewhere.

We receive two to three of these notices a year from the school and I basically ignore them now except for a check or two on the kids' heads. They know not to share hats and the usual drill, but you never know — some kids are always in such close proximity with each other. It's the head-to-head contact that really spreads lice, not clothing or other personal items. According to the Centers for Disease Control and Prevention (CDC), it is uncommon to get lice from the sharing of hats, combs or hairbrushes.[7]

The previous year, I received an email from the mom of a child who had come over to play at our house and who had lice. She had written to warn us that he had it during the visit. I immediately went into lice-checking mode, mentally tracking where he had been. In the car — check the headrests! In the house — check the... Well, I guess just check the children, since that was going to be the source of infestation, not the pile of Lego.

The "Head Lice Letter" included instructions for what to do if your child had lice, which was quite handy, and came from the school nurse's office, which really was just a form letter from the Seattle Public School District. I was impressed to see that their first recommendation for treating the hair was to choose non-toxic products and use a lice comb. It did mention chemical products to kill the lice and nits, but it was also careful to note that these products do not always kill all the lice and nits and you still needed to comb and pick them out. I was impressed, because even the CDC focused on pediculicides (potentially toxic pesticides) rather than a non-toxic treatment.[8]

At the time of receiving that email warning of a head lice invasion, I did a bit of research and the most effective way of getting rid of lice was, not too surprisingly, a lice comb. Some of the non-toxic shampoos could help make it easier to use the comb and remove the lice but, ultimately, pouring pesticides on your child's head was not the answer and had health consequences that shouldn't be taken lightly. However, I completely understood the gut reaction to any kind of personal infestation with an "Off! Now!" attitude and throwing caution to the wind just to be rid of it. My head itched just thinking about it.

However, most chemical pesticides are used because they are perceived as being a quick, low-energy fix and, more importantly, effective. But all those quick fixes were also toxic and not all were effective. Lice-killing shampoos were no different. It took work to get rid of an infestation and, since you are dealing with your child's head, it's even more important to be careful.

The CDC stated that, "The drugs used to treat lice are insecticides and can be dangerous if they are misused or overused" and they recommended a second application only if necessary or under certain circumstances. Over-the-counter lice shampoos contain permethrin or pyrethrins, both of which are neurotoxin pesticides. Pyrethrin is an extract of the chrysanthemum flower and is generally regarded as safe to use. Permethrin is a synthetic version of pyrethrin. Unfortunately, depending on where you live in the country, the "super lice" in your area may be resistant to one or both chemicals due to overuse. Additionally, permethrin is not approved for kids under the age of two and synthetic pyrethroids such as permethrin have been found to be endocrine disruptors as well.

The more commonly prescribed lice shampoos contain lindane, which is a known carcinogen and a suspected endocrine disruptor.

The EPA lists it as acutely toxic. Being an endocrine disruptor, which essentially means that it can disrupt hormone levels that regulate growth and impact reproductive health, is of particular concern to children since they are still developing. In situations where children have had acute lindane poisoning, it has caused permanent damage to the central nervous system.[9] A potent neurotoxin, it can also cause seizures and case-controlled research has shown a significant association between brain tumors in children and the use of lindane-containing lice shampoos.[10] This makes some sense since the CDC stated that it shouldn't be used on persons who weigh less than 110 pounds, which includes most children.

Lindane was banned from pharmaceutical use in California in 2001 and since that time no increase in difficulties in treating head lice have been reported in the state. In addition, it has been documented that there has been a marked decrease in lindane wastewater contamination in the state and a dramatic decline in lindane poisoning incidents reported to Poison Control Centers.

Finally, another prescription remedy contains malathion which isn't as effective as lindane, is less convenient (you have to leave it on for many hours) and shouldn't be used on children younger than six.

After reading all that I decided the most effective treatment was really just a very good, metal lice comb. There are a number of these products on the market and I ended up buying two — one for each child. I figured that, on the off-chance they got lice, they each had their own lice comb. His and hers. Now I understand the full implications of the phrase "nit picking." It is an arduous task that requires a tremendous amount of time but it's really the only way to safely get rid of lice. You have to use a strong comb and not the cheap plastic ones that come with some lice products. Some people swear by using tea tree oil or bergamot essential oil in shampoo with a vinegar rinse to help loosen the lice and the nits. There's also a battery-operated lice comb that zaps the lice with an electric current. Hopefully I'll never have to test that one.

Keeping the chemo out of me

My husband had started taking a chemotherapy drug about a year after his stem cell transplants to keep his cancer in check since his new immune system wasn't exactly doing its job as planned. It was an ongoing therapy that he took for three weeks, and then had one week off for his body to recover. When he first started taking it, the side effects included tiredness and stomach issues, but for the most part he didn't see the sorts of side effects most people think of when you say "chemotherapy," like baldness and vomiting.

The drug he was on, Revlimid (also called lenalidomide), was of a new class of drugs that targeted the cancer itself instead of all his cells like more traditional kinds of chemo. For Hank, it had been a lifesaver both before and after his stem cell transplants and had helped bring the number of cancer cells in his bone marrow down to .4 g/dl. At least, that's where he was in September, at the beginning of the project.

Revlimid can cause some unsavory side effects, though, like low blood cell counts as well as deep vein thrombosis (which my husband did get when he was first on it) and pulmonary embolism, both of which are blood clots that can do some severe damage. Revlimid gets a little bit of slack even though it's a derivative of thalidomide, which can cause severe birth defects, yet it has essentially saved and continues to save my husband's life. I am still disappointed that people want to take this drug off the market, harking back to the "thalidomide babies" from the 1960s, born from women who were taking the drug as an antiemetic. Nowadays it's not used on pregnant women for morning sickness, of course.

Today, Celgene (the manufacturer) goes a little crazy in making sure that patients taking the drug can in no way become pregnant or impregnate anyone else. Each month, before being dispensed the drug, we had to fill out a survey questioning my husband's ability to get pregnant or make someone else pregnant. It was a little tedious, but I could see why they did it. Patient education on something that was so toxic to a fetus was necessary.

The fact that it stayed in your system for four weeks after you stopped taking it was relevant as well. Well, to me, that is. If I had unprotected sex with my husband (who, due to a vasectomy and total body irradiation, is a low candidate for producing a thalidomide baby even if he wanted to), I was potentially exposed to this drug as well. I did a phone consultation with one of the providers at Celgene about the risks and, really, the problem was that they did not know what the effects were on the recipient.

In fact, the packaging stated, "You must use a latex condom, even if you have had a vasectomy (surgery that prevents a man from causing a pregnancy), every time you have sexual contact with a female who is pregnant or able to become pregnant while you are taking lenalidomide and for 4 weeks after your treatment." Frankly I think they just didn't want to take any chances. In any case, we continued to follow the directions as prescribed to prevent my possible exposure to another toxin.

Of epidemic proportions

This cancer I had never heard of up until three years prior to writing this book seemed to be coming out of the woodwork like crazy and people right and left were telling me that so-and-so was just diagnosed with multiple myeloma or that they had an uncle or a cousin with it. On one hand, I have to admit it was sort of comforting to know my husband wasn't the only one being hit by this dreadful disease, but on the other, it really pissed me off to see that the rates of diagnosis were on the rise. And it was clearly not from just a genetic predisposition.

A few weeks into the project, I was at my massage therapist's office, yakking about something or other, when she cut me off and asked rather solemnly, "Your husband has multiple myeloma, right?" I could tell this wasn't going to be the most relaxing massage I had ever experienced. It turned out that her close friend's brother had just been diagnosed with multiple myeloma and had gone into renal failure and died. It all happened so quickly, they didn't really know what was going on. Like my husband, he was diagnosed at 38 and, just like my husband, it all started with intense back pain. He had been seeing a physical therapist, just like my husband, when he started having other health problems and was finally diagnosed with multiple myeloma. He very quickly went into renal failure (not uncommon in myeloma patients) and died. He was survived by a wife and a six-month-old baby.

It pained me no end to hear stories like these, and especially one that so paralleled our own experience. I was hesitant to tell my husband about it, but I thought he might find some comfort in knowing about this other family, particularly because it showed how lucky we were. Things could have turned out that way for us as well, but didn't.

Foundations for autism

In spite of the plethora of theories on the causes, no one really knows what is at the root of autism. There is no silver bullet solution that, if we removed one thing from a fetus's, baby's or child's environment, would solve the problem. There are a number of suspected agents, but I firmly believe that it is a combination of genetic predisposition and environmental factors that tips these kids over the edge into abnormal neural development.

One extreme example of toxin exposure to kids is that Inuit women have such high levels of PCBs in their breast milk that it would be categorized as hazardous waste by the Food and Drug Administration (FDA) if they were evaluating it for human consumption.[11] This high level has more to do with the fact that more toxins end up in the Arctic due to airflow patterns, but it does raise the question that if the mother is carrying a large body burden of toxins, how much is she passing on to the child—not just through breast milk, but also in utero—and what effect does it have on the developing brain?

Most chemical substances have been shown to be anywhere from 3 to 10 times more toxic to fetuses and newborns than to adults. And by the time you are six months old, you have already received 30% of your lifetime toxic load of chemicals. With PCBs, it only takes five parts per billion in a mother's blood to cause permanent brain damage to a fetus.

One study also showed the relationship between common food additives and interference with the normal development of nerve cells.[12] The combination of these additives had up to seven times greater neurotoxic effects on nerve cell growth than when applied individually. Additives like monosodium glutamate (MSG), aspartame and artificial colorants (quinoline yellow and brilliant blue) are what shows up in a child's bloodstream after your average snack and a drink. In 1985, the medical journal *The Lancet* reported a study where 79% of hyperactive children improved when artificial colorings and flavorings were eliminated from their diet.[13]

Children who live in homes with vinyl floors, which can emit phthalates, are more likely to have autism, according to research by Swedish and U.S. scientists published in May 2010. This study of Swedish children was among the first to find an apparent connection between an environmental chemical and autism. Not too shockingly, the scientists were surprised by their findings.[14] If vinyl flooring is increasing the risk of autism, what other chemicals out there are contributing to not only autism but also ADHD?

Cluing in on ADHD

"Henry, you need to sit up. Henry, you need to get off the floor. Please be quiet. Henry, you're hurting me, please get out from under the chair."

When my son began kindergarten it became painfully obvious that he had ADHD, particularly when he was compared with other kids his age. Up to that point, he had been in a mixed-year Montessori preschool where the vast majority of kids were several years younger. There were only two other students in his preschool who were the same age as him and one had behavioral issues as well, so it was hard to tell how much was due to age and how much was his own inability to sit quietly.

The above scene played out at the introduction night before the first day of kindergarten, when all the students and parents got a chance to meet the teacher and see where the students' desks were. It was also a time for the teacher to explain to the parents her expectations as well as some administrative details. Henry was too agitated to sit at his desk, so he sat on my lap on the sidelines of the class, along with the other parents and siblings. The rest of his classmates were sitting at their desks, listening to the teacher and, for the most part, paying attention.

There were a few other students who were fidgeting, but they were nothing compared to Henry. He spent the entire time bucking around on my lap, sliding onto the floor, crawling under my chair and generally making it nearly impossible for me to pay attention to anything the teacher was saying. We ended up leaving after about 20 minutes since his agitation just kept escalating. I chalked it up to his anxiety about starting a new school, but I left feeling very frustrated and, frankly, quite embarrassed. Since Henry never wanted to play with other kids his age, I never had a social yardstick to use to know how far off the range of normal he truly was.

It wasn't just his social awkwardness and immaturity; it was his lack of being "there." I never considered him to have ADHD, mostly because when he's interested in something he can concentrate on it for *hours*, barely moving a muscle. I always believed that his ignoring us when he wasn't interested in something was just his way of letting us know that he wasn't, well, interested. I think I was really just ignoring the symptoms because most of the time, when he wasn't quietly obsessing over something he liked, he was, mentally, somewhere else. I used to always describe it as my son being in an "unreachable place." Because it was, truly, like talking to someone whose mind was on another planet.

After that initial assessment back in preschool, I decided to take him to a neurologist to get a professional opinion, since I suspected he had Tourette's Syndrome, commonly referred to as Tourette's, and to get some help. Henry exhibited the same fidgety behavior during his appointment as he had on the kindergarten meeting night. He spent the time climbing on and off the exam table and mostly ignoring the doctor's questions.

Our neurologist was the one who pointed out his attention deficits. Having ADHD (which is a neurobehavioral disorder characterized by the inability to pay attention, accompanied by hyperactivity and impulsivity) and being labeled as such can be quite an issue at school.[15] If the student exhibits disruptive behavior it's very likely that the teachers will suggest medication. We didn't have this experience at our school, mostly because it was decided, with our neurologist, to not put Henry on a traditional ADHD stimulant medication. This is strictly because, in patients with tic disorders, the stimulant made the tics much worse.

Instead, we decided to try a medication that was found to reduce the tics in Tourette's patients and also had the added benefit of calming down the ADHD. It was essentially a blood pressure medication that cleared the bloodstream quickly, so he took it twice a day. I can't say that it completely reduced his inattention and impulsivity—those were still there—but it was better and, as he got older, we decreased the dosage.

However, reports from school still showed that Henry was incredibly disruptive in class, upward of several times an hour, even after being on medication for three years. The teachers knew of Henry's issues and, by then, he was on an individual education plan (IEP) for his behavioral problems, mostly related to social issues and disruptive behavior. At the beginning of this project, we were still decreasing the dosage slowly to see if he still needed it. Our neurologist first mentioned that most kids taper off it after being on it for a few years.

Most people shudder at the idea of putting their children on medication for behavioral problems, but I'd argue that those parents don't know what it's like to watch their child struggle and suffer without help. No one castigates the parent who dutifully administers medication for diabetes or other childhood illnesses, but the same isn't true for behavioral problems. Oftentimes the parent is blamed for the child's behavior, being accused of bad parenting, or for wanting to have an "easier" child to deal with. I'm sure there are some cases of that, but overall, most parents would love to not have to medicate their children so they can function closer to normal. Medication is not a cure by any means — the behaviors are still there, just reduced.

What does ADHD have to do with toxins? Well, there have been a number of theories and studies done on the effects of environmental toxins influencing the increase in ADHD in individuals, most notably artificial flavoring, preservatives and coloring as mentioned above. Additionally, synthetic food additives have been connected to irritability, aggressiveness and excitability.[16]

While my son definitely exhibits all of these behaviors, his neurodevelopmental problems extend beyond just external inputs. We eliminated much of the artificial food agents from his diet, mostly because I generally just didn't buy those sorts of products and I couldn't say that I had seen much of a reduction in his behavioral problems compared to when he was eating or drinking the occasional "offending" chemicals. I could see how they could potentially push an otherwise neurologically normal child into behavior problems, but it just didn't seem to be the case for Henry. At any rate, I still kept these chemicals out of his diet as much as possible.

Sticky situation

Years ago, I remember reading about the dangers of heating Teflon and other nonstick-coated pans too high as the gas produced was enough to kill people's pet birds. Talk about a canary in the coal mine. Not only are birds affected by this gas, but people are as well. Symptoms of polymer fume fever, caused by the chemical polytetrafluoroethylene (PTFE) off-gassing into perfluorooctanoic acid (PFOA), include flu-like symptoms that last for several days. Although rare, more severe toxic effects like pulmonary edema, pneumonitis and death can also occur.

PFOA is a relatively nasty chemical in that it persists indefinitely in both the environment and the body. It is a known toxicant and is carcinogenic and has been found, pervasively, in the blood of humans. An ongoing study of people exposed to this chemical in the area around the Dupont facility (the creator of Teflon) to determine if PFOA leads to an increased risk of disease will be completed in 2011. For now, it is known to raise cholesterol and uric acid levels, but adverse health effects have yet to be proven — which was the case with most of the chemicals I was trying to avoid.

Off-gassing occurs when the pans are heated too high, but studies have shown that off-gassing temperatures can be reached very quickly even on a medium setting. In most circumstances, the off-gassing may not be enough to cause any noticeable problems (like the symptoms of polymer fume fever or worse), but there's still a risk of breathing in those fumes. Most people don't heed the warning to never heat a nonstick pan higher than medium. And that's not even mentioning cooking and eating from a scratched nonstick pan. The manufacturers claim that there is no harm in digesting bits of nonstick coating, but I knew I didn't want a steady diet of it.

My husband, who was far more worried about the coating than I was, refused to cook on Teflon-coated pans for years. In fact, we didn't have any nonstick pans for about five years, preferring our anodized stainless steel, aluminum-core All Clad set as well as enamel and cast iron cookware. It wasn't until my brother-in-law came to visit a few years ago and was horrified at the fact that we didn't have a Teflon-coated skillet that things changed. He complained while he was here and, shortly after his visit, we received in the mail an All Clad nonstick skillet. Presumably for the next time he visited. This was sent in spite of both of us saying we didn't want anything nonstick.

This new Teflon-coated skillet sat in the kitchen cabinet for a year before I finally decided to give it a try. I convinced myself that, by making sure I never heated it above medium, it "should be fine." I used it for making eggs, which wasn't very often, but my husband still refused to use it. It wasn't until I learned how to actually cook eggs properly in our stainless steel skillet that I stopped using it. You really just don't need nonstick if you know what you are doing and have the right equipment.

The funny thing is that, although my husband adamantly refused to use our Teflon skillet, he had no problem using all the other nonstick baking and cooking items in the house. My husband is a fantastic baker and bakes a lot—more than my waistline can generally handle. We had gone out of our way to avoid Teflon in frying pans, but we didn't really notice how ubiquitous nonstick chemicals were, as well as the inherent danger of heating them in the oven, under the broiler and on the stove top. Our nonstick items included our Bundt cake, tube and pizza pans, my beloved Zojirushi rice cooker, our Crock-Pot slow cooker, muffin tins and bread pans.

What *is* known is that more than half of all cookware sold in the U.S. has some sort of nonstick coating. What we also know is that every single one of us has Teflon in our blood in varying levels, with children having higher concentrations than adults. We may not have any definitive studies pointing to negative health effects yet, but if it is making its way into the bodies of humans worldwide and it stays, locked in our fat stores, I was certain I didn't want any more of it added in there.

So, where did that leave us in this project? Pretty much the only safe surfaces we could cook on were cast iron, Pyrex glass and stainless steel. Fortunately, we had plenty of those items. The hard part was avoiding some of the pans for baking as we didn't have alternatives. I went back to cooking rice old-school-style—on the stove.

A frictionless surface

But it wasn't just our cooking and baking ware that was full of PTFE. It covers the inside of candy wrappers and chip bags; it coats our fabric, furniture, carpets, clothing, the lining of microwave popcorn bags and much more. It's almost impossible to avoid since most new products tout the convenience of stain resistance and wrinkle resistance and the benefits of things not sticking to each other. Well, in many cases, I think it's okay for things to stick together when the alternative is still quite unknown.

All of our furniture is leather. We didn't have fabric chairs or furniture, but I bet if we did they'd be coated in some sort of stain-resistant chemical. We did, however, have wrinkle-free and water-repellant clothing and I never really gave much thought to what made the fabric stain resistant, water repellant or wrinkle free.

Gore-Tex and other water-repellant fabrics all have some form of Teflon-like chemical involved, unless they're made out of PVC, which has its own issues. Gore-Tex and other barrier-style waterproof and breathable fabrics are made of Teflon. The coating (usually called something like DWR for durable water repellent finish) is made from some form of fluoropolymers. You can even buy a spray for your clothes to help "refresh" lost water repellency. I like to think of it as liquid Teflon. In any case, I'd hate to breathe that stuff in and, as far as I can tell from the can, there's no warning against inhaling it.

All of my coats and jackets, except the leather ones, have some sort of DWR finish on them. Of course, I also have one with Gore-Tex in addition to the DWR for a Teflon double whammy. I really only used it if it was snowing out or raining like crazy and I was outside dealing with our backyard chickens. I continued using my water-resistant coats during the project because of their utility, especially in Seattle. I couldn't imagine getting chicken poop and dirt all over my leather coats and not being able to wash them. Plus, heading out in the pouring rain in an expensive leather jacket is just plain stupid.

Another option would have been to get a boiled wool coat, which is naturally water repellant. Again, the ease of cleaning it after doing "farm" chores was not reasonable and I still would have fallen back on the Gore-Tex/DWR coat. My other coats all have a DWR finish on them and still got a ton of use. I really just couldn't get around the problem. On days when it wasn't raining or at times when I wasn't dealing with chicken poop, which were far and few between, I wore my leather coats.

It was the same issue with stain- and wrinkle-resistant fabric. Since I was working from home I didn't need to be wearing anything too presentable, so avoiding those types of fabrics was easy. I only had a few wrinkle-resistant shirts and I generally didn't wear them very often anyway, so their avoidance, whether or not I was going in to work, wasn't going to be a problem. In any case, I put them in the donation pile.

My husband, on the other hand, wears wrinkle-resistant clothing every day at work. He had ordered a bunch of new shirts for his birthday in early October at the start of this project and didn't think twice about the wrinkle-resistant problem. I could have made him return them and get "regular" shirts without fancy coatings on them, but that just meant that he'd need to do a whole lot more ironing or, rather, I'd be doing a whole lot of ironing to make up for it. Personally, I could avoid them, but I didn't feel comfortable making my husband switch out his whole work wardrobe.

So, short of wearing oiled canvas, boiled wool or leather coats, avoiding the Teflon-like coatings was difficult when it came to outdoor apparel for the entire family. I wore alternatives when I could, but for the most part, I was still exposed to Teflons when it rained heavily and made do with fleece when cleaning out the chicken coop unless it was pouring out.

Coal tar cake with a side of Teflon

My husband's birthday was at the beginning of October and, since he's Mr. Baker, he made his own birthday cake. I know this sounds like cruel and unusual punishment, but he loves to bake so it's really just an excuse for him to have an opportunity to bake whatever cake he feels like making. This year he was hell-bent on making a Velvet Chocolate Cake from a new baking book we got over the summer. We had spent three weeks on the east coast visiting family, ending with a week in Greenwich Village, about a block from the café and bakery Amy's Bread. We went there to sample the goods at least once, if not twice, a day and I ate the most amazing chocolate cake known to man. I think I gained about 10 pounds from that leg of the trip, but it was well worth it. Amy's has a couple of cookbooks and so, in order to continue the gluttony from home, we picked one of them up and my husband had been making cakes out of it since then.

Unfortunately, the particular recipe he was looking at for his birthday required the use of red food coloring. In the past he's just used high-quality baking food coloring, but I didn't know what its chemical origins were. This time around we discussed what the options were. Quite a few red food colorings, which are listed in the ingredients as carmine, come from cochineal insects. I'm fine with eating bugs since it's better than eating something derived from coal tar, which is what many yellow and red food colorings are made of. You can get naturally derived food colorings for pretty much every color you need—green made from seaweed, red made from beets, yellow from turmeric and the like.

It got a little more confusing when we looked into the artificial food colorings, all of which were considered safe to eat but are banned in some European countries for a variety of potential health issues. For example, FD&C Red #3 is a suspected carcinogen and is commonly used in food. It is also derived from coal tar or, more specifically, erythrosine, which has been shown to cause thyroid tumors in high doses. In addition, new studies have shown a potential link between artificial food coloring agents and aggravated ADD and ADHD symptoms in both the general population and those individuals already affected.

Over the years, we've mostly switched to natural foods that have few artificial colorings in them, although there are still some foods the kids eat that I'm sure use them. I have tried to limit the most outrageously colored foods because I had heard of the link between dyes and hyperactivity, which we didn't need any more of in this house. But there were many food products out there that contained them. In other words, the use of artificial colors was a lot more insidious than you would think and looking at ingredient lists is imperative if you want to avoid them. Oftentimes packaging leads you to believe something is a lot more benign than it is.

For example, just looking in our kitchen cabinet, we had a box of Sunkist Fruit Gems which purported to be "naturally flavored soft fruit candies, made with real fruit juice" with no mention of how they were colored. It was easy to make the leap from "natural and real" to the assumption that the colors were also natural. But according to the ingredients, the candies contained FD&C Yellow #5 and #6, Red #3 and #40 and Blue #1. That's a serving of tartrazine (from the Yellow #5) and erythrosine (from the Red #3), both derived from coal tar, both suspected of health implications and both banned in some countries.

For his cake, my husband was uninterested in using naturally derived food colorings from plants, mainly because he had read that they tend to impart a particular flavor to what you are baking. Red Velvet Cake that tastes like beets wasn't really something he was interested in making. There were other options. Red can also be derived from paprika, red grape skins and other natural foods, but these alternative options can be expensive, harder to come by and require special ordering ahead of time — not the day before you make the cake. I was hoping to find the bug- or beet-based ones, because they are commonly used.

Looking up the ingredients in the artificial color Allura Red (which we had in the kitchen), I found lead, arsenic, mercury, cadmium and other heavy metals.[17] I compared that to the ingredient list for Nature's Flavors liquid Natural Red Food Color made from beets and the full ingredient list was, drum roll please, water and beets.[18] I was sure that the artificial color, which was far cheaper, also had better merits in terms of suspension in a cake batter and probably spread better and didn't bleed and all that, but I was also fairly sure that a dose, however small, of heavy metals in a cake just wasn't very appetizing.

Another issue that came up in regards to my husband's birthday cake was that I thought all we had in the kitchen for baking were nonstick cake pans. Things were starting to look pretty bad for my consumption of any of this cake at that point. Between the food coloring and the nonstick pans, I figured there was no way I was going to get a piece of non-toxic birthday cake. I had forgotten that my husband had recently purchased new cake pans, the Fat Daddio's anodized aluminum cake pans that are made with brushed aluminum. Anodizing aluminum seals the pan while making it scratch resistant and ensures that there's no cross-contamination or leaching of aluminum into foods. In looking at their product line and querying the company directly, I found out that many of their products do not use a nonstick coating, so we ended up replacing many of our other pans with their product line during the project.

In anticipation of cake baking, my husband and I headed out to Home Cake Decorating Supply Co. in the Maple Leaf neighborhood of Seattle, where we've gone many times in the past for birthday cake-making supplies. It's a great little store that sells pretty much everything you could possibly need for making cakes at home, although the place looks a bit like a tornado hit it. It's packed full of items in a very small space with little organization about it, but once you figure out where to look for something, you're sure to unearth a gem. We've purchased gel paste food coloring there in the past and I didn't remember seeing any alternatives for natural food coloring, but the place is such a mess it was possible that it was hidden somewhere and I just didn't see it.

I chalked it up to wishful thinking that they would have any alternatives but, of course, all they carried were AmeriColor gel pastes and powdered artificial food colorings. I snuck a peek at the ingredients and all their various shades of red included FD&C Red #3 and Yellow #5. After going over the basic issues with artificial food colorings with him, my husband bought the AmeriColor Red-Red food coloring anyway.

While we were checking out, I spoke to the owner, Griel, about whether or not they carried natural food coloring. She explained that she didn't want to get into supplying them for a few reasons. The first, most obvious one was that the natural colorants didn't perform as well and she didn't want to deal with customers returning the products, unhappy with the results. The second and equally important issue was the cost. She suggested that other local stores like Whole Foods were carrying natural food colorants that were $40 for a small amount and people were unimpressed by them. Having looked them up online beforehand I thought the cost was a bit of an exaggeration. Natural food coloring usually runs about $15, which is still quite a bit more than the $2.50 we paid for the Red-Red.

After leaving the store, I suggested we head over to Whole Foods to see what they had on offer since it was down the street. I also suggested that Hank could make one layer with the artificial coloring and one with the natural coloring to see not only what the flavor difference was, but also what the performance was. It sounded like a great experiment and, since I hadn't yet done my initial lab tests, trying out a little Red #3 and Yellow #5 cocktail wasn't going to hurt just yet.

Unfortunately, the only food coloring Whole Foods carried was a liquid food coloring that was more appropriate for beverages and icing than for baked goods. It even stated on the bottle that "natural colors may not be heat stable and may change their original color at high temperatures." As I suspected, it was only $13 or so. The brand they carried was Select and their red was made out of hibiscus extract and beet powder extract. I was game to give it a try, of course, but I knew it wasn't appropriate for what my husband was making so we ended up just getting the artificial coloring. I didn't want him ending up with a weirdly gray cake.

I had the chance to eat some of the cake as my initial screening blood tests were scheduled for the day after his birthday party. We both agreed it wasn't very good and, frankly, it wasn't worth ingesting the food coloring. It was a hell of a lot of trouble to go to just for a cake.

Falling for candles

Fall in Seattle is my favorite season. Usually. This particular year, though, the weather had been less than stellar—we had a very cold summer and the fall was shaping up to be not too much better with a lot of clouds and drizzle. Generally, September is the last month of the year where we have any chance of a few clear skies, the kind where you can actually see the sky rather than the low, dark overhang of clouds that starts up in October and lasts until April. October is also when we start losing our daylight at an astonishing rate. And that's when we start busting out the candles.

Since we are so far north, we get spoiled during the summer where it can stay light out until 9 and 10 PM. But we get paid back on the other end where, by the end of fall, it's dark out at 4 PM. Lighting candles doesn't exactly help fight the darkness, it just adds a lot more ambience to an otherwise dreary evening. And, since lighting candles during the summer is just plain ridiculous, by the time October rolls around, I'm generally champing at the bit to light some during our Sunday family dinners.

Sunday family dinners have been a tradition in our family since 2007 where, at the very least, my mom comes over to a full sit-down dinner and, if other family members are available or are in town, they have an open invitation to come as well. I like the regularity of it, it helps start the week off right and it also gives us an excuse to prepare a larger meal. Oftentimes, it is a roasted organic chicken that I can then make stock out of the next day and stretch the leftovers out for a few more meals.

Planning for the dinner starts a few days in advance. I generally focus on the dinner and my husband works the dessert. It's the only day of the week that we sit at our formal dining table in the dining room (rather than the table in the kitchen), so it feels special. We set a formal table and the kids get to drink milk or juice from wine glasses and, of course, during the darker months, we light candles for the center of the table.

There are a number of candle material choices, the most common ones being made of paraffin, which is an inexpensive petroleum waste by-product. When burned, paraffin emits benzene and toluene and breathing in its smoke is just as dangerous as breathing in secondhand cigarette smoke. Even many candles labeled as beeswax contain a lot of paraffin because it is cheap. Gel candles are also made of petroleum and consist of synthetic hydrocarbons with some butylated hydroxyl toluene thrown in for good measure. Needless to say, burning and breathing in the atomized particles of these contaminants isn't good for one's health.

Newer on the market are soy candles or vegetable oil–based ones that burn a lot cleaner than petroleum-based ones and are recommended if you want healthier indoor air and still want to burn candles, but I prefer beeswax by far. The cleanest-burning candles you can buy are ones made from 100% organic beeswax with an organic cotton wick. Beeswax is purported to help "clean" the air because it emits negative ions. I'm still not sure if I buy the ionization business, but I do know that, even if beeswax candles don't clean the air, they are cleaner burning than anything else out there (except for not lighting candles in the first place, of course).

In all cases, where the candles are manufactured is important because there still is some risk of buying one with a lead wick. Lead hasn't been used in the manufacture of wicks in the U.S. for decades, but it is still possible to buy one if it came from overseas. Burning wicks with lead or a lead core can result in unsafe levels of lead in the air and consistent exposure to lead candles can significantly impact the lead levels in the human body.

I'm not a huge fan of scented candles, and I particularly don't like burning scented ones in close proximity to where we are eating. It's hard to taste your food when you are overwhelmed by "Autumn Spice" or "Cranberry Orange" scented candles. The bigger issue with scented candles is how they are fragranced. Much like other products with synthetic fragrances, the full ingredients aren't listed and are exempt from disclosure since they are considered to be a proprietary blend.

Usually this means that the ingredient listing "fragrance" tends to be a catch-all for more dubious ingredients, and almost all of them contain toluene and phthalates. Toluene can cause nervous system damage and is often contaminated with small amounts of benzene, which is a known cause of leukemia, while phthalates are known endocrine disruptors.[19] A single fragrance can be made up of more than 100 different chemicals. Of the chemicals found in synthetic fragrances that have been tested, almost 30% are considered to be toxic.[20]

Occasionally, I do like a scented candle. I just make sure that it's made out of beeswax and uses essential oils for fragrance instead of synthetic chemicals. And if there are any colorants in the scented candles (the unscented beeswax ones are generally a natural color), I make sure the dyes used are also natural and not synthetic.

And, as much as I love burning a thousand candles for the effect, I don't for a number of reasons. The first is that it's expensive and I don't get that much more out of it, but the more important reason is indoor air quality. Although burning 100% organic beeswax candles with cotton wicks is far better than burning a scented paraffin candle with a lead wick, I'm still burning something and that small amount of smoke can build up and isn't good for the lungs. I still had some questionable candles in our possession during this project, mostly tea candles made out of paraffin. Every time I run low on beeswax candles I'm tempted to burn the loads of tea candles we have, particularly for Halloween lighting, and I give in and convince myself that a few little candles won't hurt. This fall and winter, however, I made sure I stuck with only the beeswax or skipped them altogether.

Mammograms and mercury, oh my!

When my husband was diagnosed with cancer in September of 2007, I got so caught up in his health care, trying not only to keep him alive but also to help him reduce his symptoms, that I couldn't bring myself to go to the doctor. Between the chemotherapy treatments and the ensuing year and a half of transplants and post-transplant visits, I couldn't handle going to the doctor for an annual exam because I couldn't mentally handle it if they found something wrong with me, too.

I know this sounds horribly ridiculous and possibly negligent, but prior to that I was very diligent about going to the doctor every year and making sure everything was in tip-top shape. Now getting a suspicious pap result or finding a lump would have completely thrown me over the edge. I still went in for dental visits, flu shots and if I had something else going on, like the strep my son brought home from school, but I avoided the general physical lest they find something unusual.

I finally bit the bullet after the kids started back to school and my schedule became flexible with writing this book and went in for an "annual" exam. It was the basic physical with blood pressure test, listening to the heart and lungs, with a breast and pelvic exam and pap smear. All were normal, fortunately. It had been three and a half years.

Because my husband has a compromised immune system, all of us need to get the flu vaccine each year so I asked for and got the seasonal flu vaccination during my exam. The flu shot I got was the multishot vial of flu vaccine that contained thimerosal as a preservative. Thimerosal contains ethyl mercury and, since I got the shot before doing the lab tests for heavy metals, I suspected it might have some impact on the results. I later asked Dr. Hibbs (the doctor working on my body burden labs) about whether or not this could affect the results of the mercury testing, and he explained that it "would have a very small effect, lessening rapidly as time passes." On one hand I was worried that getting the shot would potentially skew the results of my mercury testing but, on the other hand, getting annual immunizations was part of life and should be included, rather than avoided, in a "snapshot" of the contaminants in my system.

I was surprised to learn that the 2010–11 influenza vaccine was a combo that included the A/H1N1 strain in additional to the other seasonal strains. The kids and I got the "swine" flu aka H1N1 the previous year the natural way (my husband got the vaccine so he missed out) so I already had immunity to it. I would have preferred to have gotten the thimerosal-free vaccine, but it's hard to find the single-shot dosage that is free of the preservative. The FluMist nasal spray vaccine doesn't contain thimerosal and I had it many years ago, but we can't use the FluMist now because it contains a live, attenuated (weakened) virus and it isn't recommended if you live with individuals with a weakened immune system.

Later, after I got the vaccination, I called the doctor's office to find out the name of the manufacturer of the flu vaccination they gave me because you can find out all sorts of interesting things online, like the amount of mercury in a dose. The woman who answered the phone kind of groaned at my question, giving the impression that I was one of *those* patients, but she was able to find out. Sanofi Pasteur was the manufacturer and, based on the information on their website, the dose of the FluZone shot that I received had 25 mcg of ethyl mercury.[21] How did this compare to say, eating some fish like tuna? It was about the equivalent of eating a can of light tuna but, since it was ethyl mercury and not methyl mercury (like in tuna), it stayed in the blood for a shorter amount of time.

I would have loved to have gotten the single-dose, thimerosal-free vaccines for the kids, particularly for Henry. There has been a tremendous amount of controversy over the years regarding thimerosal vaccines and the incidence of autism. To date, no studies have shown a definitive link between the two, but the idea that kids on the autism range are more sensitive to processing mercury makes me more cautious about introducing more into his system—particularly since several studies have shown that, due to exposure to thimerosal in utero, the incidence of tics was increased.[22] I didn't know what kind of impact thimerosal could potentially have as a single dose via a vaccine, but we certainly didn't need to accentuate any tics or behavioral issues.

In the end, we couldn't get the preservative-free vaccine, but we still got the kids vaccinated. Both of them have had them in the past and I haven't seen any difference behaviorally or otherwise and this year was no different. Henry was unaffected by the vaccine and the benefits to my husband were incentive enough to risk it.

Now that I'm of a certain age, the topic of mammograms came up during that annual exam. I had read a bunch of conflicting information on mammograms before that visit, mostly revolving around the number of false positives and the medical machinery one gets trapped in if something does show up. My doctor did mention that other countries, Western European countries mainly, don't start doing mammograms until women are 50.

I asked her what the recommendation was for getting mammograms and she said that it's every year starting at 40 and if you have three clear years, then you can do it every other year. This sounded like a lot to me, given the fact that they didn't seem tremendously accurate and that I knew of women who had something show up on a mammogram and freaked out over it and got a ton of treatment and all the while they weren't sure if treatment was necessary in the first place.

There are other diagnostic tools, but they are expensive or have higher amounts of radiation and I was in a quandary about what to do. I didn't have any history of breast cancer in my family, only took low-dose birth control pills briefly, breastfed for two years and have no history of anything suspicious. My doctor was in the middle of suggesting good choices of where to get a mammogram done when I told her I wanted to think about it. She was kind of shocked, I think, and then stated, "Well, you did just turn 40." It was like I was a ticking time bomb. And we left it at that.

Newer guidelines suggest that screening mammograms should be done every two years beginning at age 50 for women at average risk of breast cancer. But the Mayo Clinic still recommends screening mammograms from age 40. So, what the heck are we supposed to do with this conflicting information?

I discussed the issue with my husband, who knows all about cancer and its happy fun times as well as the effects of false positive results. He suggested I take her advice and get a baseline mammogram, and if anything shows up, ignore it and get tested again in a year. I told him that's all fine and good, but there's no way anyone can comfortably ignore a potentially cancerous tumor once you know it's there, even if it's just a spot. You're going to want to aspirate it and there's a high probability you're going to fall into the cogs of treatment.

Not to mention that increased exposure to radiation increases the risk of cancer and compression can increase the risk of cancer cells spreading if, in fact, they already do exist in the breast. I didn't decide much of anything at the time, because I was wary of increased exposure to radiation and would rather hold off on it. The average dose of radiation from a mammogram is equal to about two months of natural background radiation.[23] A few people recommended that I look into getting a thermogram done instead, but I really needed to do some research on what it was, how the two compared and what the other options there were out there.

PART 3

The Baseline

Testing, testing, 1-2-3…

I realized when I finally got scheduled to do the baseline blood work and urine testing for my body burden testing that it had been seven months since I first contacted Metametrix about their environmental toxicity test panels. Since then, I had worked with a few publishers, gotten the book contract and then hunkered down in earnest to find a local physician to coordinate getting the blood draws and shipping the samples to the lab. It seemed like forever had passed when the moment finally came.

The body burden tests that I ended up actually getting done were for chlorinated pesticides, PCBs, phthalates and parabens, volatile solvents and toxic metals (whole blood and urine). There was a screw-up in getting the phthalates and parabens test kit from Metametrix so I had to go back the following week to do the urine test for that. But that just meant that I had another week of exposure to those bath and beauty products that contained them. I would have loved to have done the BPA testing as well as testing for PFOAs (nonstick chemicals), but I just couldn't find a lab that would work with individual samples.

In anticipation of the tests, I had made sure that I was using my "regular" products, but other than that, I was just going about my business as usual. The only thing that was a little different going into the tests was that I had that flu shot, which contained the preservative thimerosal (a derivative of ethyl mercury), the week before. There was a span of a day between getting my blood drawn for heavy metals and starting the urine collection for a separate heavy metals test. I purposely ate a can of tuna after the blood test and before the urine test, just to see what kind of effect it would have and if it would show a difference.

The urine collection for the heavy metals testing was definitely the most annoying of the body burden tests because I had to collect it over 24 hours. Not only did I have to remember to "harvest" my pee instead of just heading off to the bathroom, I had to make sure I didn't go anywhere for very long. It required peeing in a cup, transferring it to the collection jug and storing it in the refrigerator. Under normal circumstances, I would be more grossed out by the whole process of pee in the fridge, but we are fairly well inured to it now since my husband has to do 24-hour urine collections all the time to monitor his cancer.

One of the methods of determining the extent of Hank's cancer is to check for a certain protein in his urine. Lately, he's had to do the collection once a month (or is supposed to) as part of a research study he's doing. Except for the fact that he drinks a heck of a lot more than I do and generally needs two jugs, it's pretty much the same deal. The kids are used to making sure they don't grab the orange pee container in the fridge when they go to get the milk or the orange juice.

I was joking that we'd both be doing it at the same time and would need his and hers pee jugs in the fridge. The biggest problem for me was really the fact that the collection cup was too small and, if I waited too long in between bathroom breaks, my cup would runneth over, which was most unpleasant. Trying to balance a wobbly collection cup with a meniscus of urine up to the edge, all while trying to finish up going to the bathroom, was less than appealing. I was happy when it was over. A very minor irritation, but an irritation nonetheless.

After collecting the urine over 24 hours, I bore the indignity of processing it, which included shaking the collection jug for 30 seconds to mix it up before pouring a sample into a small vial. I made sure that the lid was on tight before embarking on this little operation. And, when I was all done, I still had 2.2 liters of pee to dispose of. After all that hard work collecting it, I wasn't about to throw out all that nitrogen, so I diluted it and used it on my trees and shrubs in the backyard for fertilizer. Fortunately, none of my neighbors were out so I didn't have to explain what I was doing.

Anyway, with the testing, I was trying to get an accurate representation of an average week, where random stuff happens. You get a flu shot, you eat some fish, you put on some sunscreen, that sort of thing. I didn't go out of my way to load up on any one contaminant, or try to avoid anything.

One thing I did do was perform a sunscreen challenge. Since I had all that tingling, numbness and muscle aching going on during the previous months, I wanted to see if the sunscreen did, in fact, have anything to do with it. When I started taking Vitamin B12 and Vitamin D supplements, the symptoms had slowly gone away but, then again, I had also stopped using the sunscreen. I wanted to make sure I wasn't missing anything, although at this point it seemed reasonable that I was having problems due to my vitamin deficiencies.

My sunscreen was loaded with parabens, so using it on my arms and legs on the days leading up to my phthalate and paraben testing seemed reasonable. I used an average amount and didn't experience any renewed neuropathy problems, so that theory was out. I had one more possible cause to investigate before I completely blamed my neuropathy on the low levels of vitamins in my system, which I ended up testing later in the project.

Stinkout

During the month of October, I was hosting a challenge on my blog to encourage people to line-dry all of their laundry. The goal was to reduce their dryer usage and, in turn, reduce their carbon footprint and save some money in the meantime. A lot of my readers air-dry their clothes during the summer, when it's warm and the weather is nice, making it an easy option. But once you head into fall, it's a lot more difficult to dry when it's constantly raining out. I had been strictly line-drying all of our laundry since the beginning of August without any issues, but as the weather became colder and it took longer to dry, some clothes started smelling a little musty. In fact, they just plain stank.

During the challenge I was also testing out a nonpetroleum, non-toxic laundry detergent (which I'll discuss later), which cleaned well, but not fantastically well. More of a "good enough" clean than anything. The combination of the wet weather, long drying times and not very effective laundry detergent left our clothes smelling a little less than fresh so I didn't mind using scented body lotions and deodorant in the lead-up to my body burden tests.

During Christmas-time the previous year I got some new perfume, Estée Lauder Cashmere Mist. I really liked it because it was subtle and not cloying. You couldn't smell it at 50 paces, only if you were up close and personal. I was going through a phase about perfumes and plunked down the money for it. However, this purchase was months before I started reading and researching about all the issues with commercial perfumes.

The Campaign for Safe Cosmetics and the Environmental Working Group had recently published a study they had commissioned on the ingredients in 17 of the top-selling perfumes and colognes. Most ingredient lists for these products were considered trade secrets and many were hidden behind the label "fragrance," as is the case with many other personal care products. In the case of perfumes, most of the products on the market contained compounds that weren't listed on the ingredient label. These ingredients included hormone disruptors and chemicals that impact the thyroid, as well as multiple chemicals that hadn't been tested for safety.[1]

Because my clothes were smelling a little wonky, I decided to whip out the Cashmere Mist. If I was going to use the perfume, now would be the time. My son, Henry, immediately declared that I stank (from the perfume) and gave himself some distance from me. Of course, he is super-sensitive to smells, having sensory issues, so I didn't take it too personally. This is the same child who will smell my pillow and blankets incessantly and declare with delight, "Smells like Mom!" so I don't think it was because of some other smell. It was just a decidedly different aroma that he wasn't used to. In any case, it worked to some degree. At least, it worked long enough for me to resolve the funky clothing problem and have the toxin testing done. Once the tests were taken, I wouldn't use anything containing "perfume" or "fragrance" or anything smacking of it for the duration of the project.

Lead and water testing

The same week that I ended up doing all the blood and urine tests for my body burden testing, I also sent in samples for testing our drinking water and the lead in our interior house paint. I worked with Anatek Labs, out of Idaho, which is a multistate-certified analytical laboratory. A number of online companies offer to test your water for under a couple of hundred dollars and they seemingly test for a huge array of contaminants, but I was leery of the quality of the results. I opted for a smaller number of contaminants from a certified lab because I believed the quality of the testing would be superior. They were on the State of Washington's online list of accredited laboratories for testing drinking water, in particular, private home well water, where lead, fluoride, arsenic, cadmium and other contaminants can be an issue.

While I was at it, I also opted to get the coliform bacteria test done as well, to see if we had not only heavy metals and the like in our water, but also fecal material. The coliform test just gives a yes/no answer as the result. If the result is "yes," then further testing can be done to determine what kind of bacteria colonies are living in your water and probably how many.

For the lead testing, I scraped a 4-inch by 4-inch chunk of paint from behind Emma's bedroom door to send in for testing. It didn't look like it had too many layers of paint between the current sky blue and the wall board. It was a pretty big chunk of paint that

I scraped off, so I was curious to see how long it would take for Emma to notice and mention the missing patch. She still hasn't.

Nail polish

About a year and a half before starting this book project, I started a second blog, titled *Green Goddess Dressing,* to specifically cover environmental issues related to fashion and beauty products. I had already been focusing a lot on beauty products on my main blog, *The Crunchy Chicken,* mostly writing about replacing commercial products with natural ones that could be made at home. Not only were the replacements considerably cheaper than manufactured ones, but you also had complete control over the ingredients when you made the products at home.

In spite of my initial enthusiasm for the new blog, I ended up posting less and less over the year. However, at the start of it, I subscribed to a few fashion magazines that occasionally featured green products, magazines like *Vogue* and *Allure.* Those subscriptions have since lapsed, mostly because I don't like wasting trees, but not before I received the Fall 2010 fashion pages in mid-summer. I also had gotten a gift certificate for Nordstrom for my birthday in July and was looking for something to purchase, so I picked up a bottle of nail polish in the "hot color" of the season. The one everyone was going to be wearing, or something like that.

It was Chanel's Paradoxal nail polish.[2] It sat on my shelf for a few months before I finally got around to looking at it, let alone trying it. Lo and behold the ingredient listing was a very scary one indeed. Most nail polishes have phased out some of the nastier ingredients that were common even just 10 years ago: toluene and formaldehyde being the big ones and phthalates being another. Revlon and OPI and some other big-name commercial brands have removed many of these ingredients so you don't have to look too hard to find a brand with fewer toxins. Not non-toxic by any means, just less toxic.

Nail polish in general is rarely going to be considered non-toxic, strictly because of the acetates and plasticizing ingredients in it. The above-mentioned bad boy, toluene, is a known toxicant and acts as a thinning agent in the polish. It is a derivate of benzene and is a volatile organic compound. The most common phthalate found in nail polish is dibutylphthalate (DBP). It acts as a plasticizing ingredient and is a potential developmental and reproductive toxin that may cause a broad range of birth defects. It has been banned for use in cosmetic products in the European Union. Last, but not least, formaldehyde works as a preservative as well as a hardener *and* it smells delicious.

More and more manufacturers — SpaRitual and OPI, for example — are getting on the bandwagon and avoiding these three chemicals but apparently Chanel still hasn't quite figured out how to substitute these ingredients and maintain the quality product they are known for. I can completely understand their not wanting to change their formulas, but having great nail color isn't worth the exposure to a couple of the first few ingredients I found listed on the bottle: ethyl acetate, phthalic anhydride, styrene and benzophenone.

Using the Environmental Working Group's Skin Deep database as my guide, I looked up these choice ingredients, starting at the end. Benzophenone was a mixed bag, earning only 2 out of 10 on the toxicity scale (with 10 being miserably toxic and 0 being safe). The research wasn't conclusive, despite some concerns about its toxicity, but anything that can be listed as a benzene gets a negative vote in my book. Styrene got a whopping 10 out of 10 for being a respiratory and immune toxicant and for showing strong evidence of human neurotoxicity as well as being an endocrine disruptor.

Moving backward, phthalic anhydride got 7 out of 10 for the same reasons as styrene minus the endocrine disruption. After further investigation, I found phthalic anhydride listed as a federal hazardous air pollutant that was identified as a toxic air contaminant in 1993. Ethyl acetate got a middling 4 for being a neurotoxin. Finally, research done by the Environmental Working Group shows that Chanel nail lacquers contain DBP (the nasty phthalate mentioned above) even though it's not listed as an ingredient.[3]

Needless to say, reading this ingredient list didn't stop me from using it the week or so before my lab tests. Again, if I was going to get an average sampling of my blood, I wasn't going to avoid a product. I wanted to represent the thousands of women falling for Chanel Paradoxal nail color that season. In fact, one of the subtests in the volatile solvents panel was specifically for styrene so I was curious to see the lab results. Once those lab tests were done, I removed the polish and kept off all nail polishes for the remainder of the five months. I never found an alternative that I felt was safe enough to use for the purposes of this project.

It's the pits

One of the first things I immediately stopped using once I had done the urine collection for the parabens and phthalates test was the antiperspirant-deodorant that I had been using. Months before I started working on this project, I had researched and written on my blog about alternatives for deodorants, mostly because there was quite a bit of buzz on environmental blogs with people opting for homemade deodorants.

My husband and I had already gone around and around on this topic before because, when he first started doing chemotherapy, he had a nasty reaction to the traditional antiperspirant-deodorant he used. It's not uncommon to have skin sensitivity when you are being bombarded by chemo, radiation and other anticancer therapies. At the time, I found a replacement product that was recommended by cancer treatment centers and rated #1 on the Environmental Working Group's Skin Deep site. It was the Crystal deodorant that relies on mineral salts and alum rather than the traditional aluminum that works as an antiperspirant to block sweat. It works by prohibiting bacterial growth. The Crystal didn't block sweat but did a fair job of keeping the smell down as long as you showered every day and didn't sweat too much. Otherwise, the stink began.

Personally, I've always been a heavy antiperspirant user. It's a family curse—we all sweat mightily and have problems with traditional products leaving stains on our clothes. This combination of genetics, bacteria and product ingredients results in a lot of ruined shirts. When I started using the Crystal a few years ago, I was pleased to find that it didn't affect my clothing and I could wear white again without the telltale yellow stains. Over the course of the last few years I had started using my old, regular antiperspirant-deodorant again, mostly due to long stretches of severe stress from dealing with some issues with Henry and Hank. I was more anxious than usual and didn't want to be any more sweaty and stinky than necessary.

About a year earlier I had also dabbled in trying a homemade deodorant which I actually liked quite a bit and preferred it to the Crystal and, for the most part, to standard antiperspirants. It didn't prevent me from sweating, which can be a problem on occasion, but if I did sweat I didn't stink, unlike with the Lady Mitchum I had been using. If I started sweating even with regular antiperspirant-deodorants I still didn't smell great.

This time around, when I dumped the Lady Mitchum after the phthalates test, I skipped the Crystal and went back to my homemade product. The only issue I had with the homemade stuff previously was with the baking soda ingredient which can be irritating and became painful to use after a while. In order to prevent this, I reworked the formula and added more of the other ingredients to offset the baking soda irritation. I wanted to avoid the reaction that I had the last time I used it and which was the reason I stopped using it in the first place. I am not the only one who has had this irritation experience and the end result after long-term use (for me, at least) was that it turned my armpits into a lovely shade of brown. Brown, thickened skin that, I realized one day while waxing my armpits, will peel off in large chunks. This, not too surprisingly, scared the crap out of me.

For this project, I felt I had the formula worked out a little better, albeit not perfectly. The recipe was a combination of corn starch (for absorption), baking soda (for odor), coconut oil and cocoa butter (as a base and for spreadability) and essential oils for a natural scent. I started off by alternating with the Crystal to prevent crusty brown pits. I had been tempted to also use the unscented Ban Roll-On that got only a toxicity rating of 1 out of 10 on the Skin Deep database, but there were still some issues with it containing aluminum which meant I only used it when I really needed to stay dry or knew I was going into a stressful situation (like a TV news interview or some such thing).

Aside from the aluminum issues (which I'll get to next), most

---

Homemade Hippie Deodorant

(This is my original recipe. Lower the amount of baking soda if you find it's irritating.)

Ingredients
- 2 Tbsp coconut oil
- 1.5 Tbsp cocoa butter
- 2 Tbsp baking soda
- 2 Tbsp corn starch
- Sandalwood and/or vanilla essential oil

While sandalwood essential oil isn't exactly sustainable, it gives the deodorant a nice smell that covers any off-putting smells your body produces and sandalwood is supposed to be antimicrobial. The cocoa butter kind of overpowers any smell in there, so if you don't like that make sure you buy deodorized cocoa butter.

Directions
Melt the oil and butter in the microwave, add in the dry ingredients, mix well and then add in the essential oil(s) one drop at a time to your liking. You can pour the cooled, but still liquid, deodorant into a clean 2.5 oz. deodorant plastic applicator for easy application and put it in the fridge to harden. Make sure the applicator is the kind with the "screw" in the middle of it. If you don't have an old applicator, you can pour it into a small wide-mouth canning jar or other small lidded container and put it in the fridge to solidify.

---

antiperspirant-deodorants have some issues with toxic ingredients, mostly from fragrances. In older studies, parabens were found in every sample of tissue taken from 20 different breast tumors. Although most deodorants and antiperspirants don't tend to use parabens in them as a preservative anymore, it's best to avoid a product with them. There is no direct link at this point suggesting that parabens cause breast cancer, but since they mimic estrogen activity in the body it's safe to say that they really should not be there in the first place and, if I can avoid them, I will. My Lady Mitchum and Ban Roll-On didn't contain parabens, but the former did have fragrance, which was mostly likely a healthy serving of phthalates instead. And both contained aluminum zirconium tetrachlorohydrex glycine and aluminum chlorohydrate respectively.

The issue with aluminum-based compounds in antiperspirants is that they also cause similar estrogen-like effects which, in turn, have the ability to promote breast cancer cell growth. Some researchers suggest that these compounds may contribute to the development of breast cancer.[4] Since it is also a known carcinogen, for the duration of the project I stuck to the alternative, aluminum-free products, except for the occasional sweat-prevention. My pits may not have always been happy about it, but I'm pretty sure my breasts were.

Tapping the tap water

Seattle purportedly has some of the best drinking water in the country, meeting all drinking water standards with no lead and low levels, if not *no* levels, of toxins. Still, people who live here tend to filter their water mostly for taste and concerns about water quality. When I compare here to other areas of the country that I've lived in and travelled through, I can't complain too much. The water here tastes pretty good, but occasionally, especially when the water reservoirs get low at the end of the summer, it tastes like a chlorine bomb. When they flush the fire hydrants, all the silt in the pipes gets stirred up and the water is rusty red and fairly undrinkable. And then there's the occasional algae problem when the water tastes like low tide on a hot day.

Our water, because it comes from protected watersheds, doesn't have some of the major contaminants that the EPA requires testing for but it has to be tested for them anyway. These include benzenes, vinyl chloride, BPA, triclosan, DEET, mercury, cadmium, perchlorate, phthalates, DDT, PCBs, atrazine and other pesticides, *E. coli* and fecal coliforms. Other interesting contaminants that can end up in the water supply (but aren't detected in ours) are chloroform, caffeine, acetaminophen, ibuprofen, nicotine, fungicides and other antibacterials used in agriculture and livestock.[5] Fortunately, none of the above have been detected in our water supply.

Even though Seattle's water is relatively toxin-free, that does not mean that metals aren't leaching from our pipes. According to Seattle Public Utilities, "[t]he majority of homes have some risk of lead contamination in water that sits in pipes for longer than 2 hours."[6] And then there's the issue of untested chemicals like chlorine and fluoride, which I'll get into in a bit.

Somewhere in between the Tolt River (where our water comes from), the reservoir where the water is treated and then tested and when it comes out of the tap there was the possibility of a difference in water quality. Getting the water analysis from Seattle Public Utilities, coupled with getting our home water tested, meant I could get a decent idea of how clean our water truly was. I worked with a lab to test for not just heavy metals and contaminants like arsenic, copper, lead, disinfectants, nitrates and cadmium, but also bacterial contaminants. The bacterial contaminants had as much to do with my own curiosity as well as human health issues, given that my husband had a compromised immune system and I had been having a lot of problems earlier in the year with gastrointestinal issues.

I knew going in to the testing that we would probably test high for copper since we had blue-green stains in the porcelain tub which are indicative of copper staining. I wasn't sure about the lead and I expected all the other contaminants to be low, given that our source water had few issues with toxicants like cadmium and arsenic. And there were other additives like chlorine and fluoride to think about too.

Holy fluorosis, Batman!

City water fluoridation programs across the United States purposefully add fluoride to the drinking water in concentrations at levels below 2 mg/L where it is thought to be beneficial to teeth and bones. The City of Seattle tested the water we get from the Tolt River and showed it to be 1.04 mg/L. Fluoride levels above 4 mg/L that are ingested for many years may result in fluorosis, which is a potentially crippling bone disorder.[7] Most recently, the recommended levels have come under debate as more children are showing signs of dental spotting due to the excess amount of fluoride exposure.

The more I read about how our water in this country came to be fluoridated, the more I realized that Americans have been the victims of an enormous health scam promulgated by the Aluminum Company of America back in the early 1940s. Silicofluoride, a toxic waste by-product of factory smokestacks, was proposed as an additive to drinking water in the *belief* that it would help prevent tooth decay. At the time, dentists, physicians and scientists were worried about adding this aluminum waste to public water and that the risk to human health far outweighed any good that would come of it.

Over the ensuing decades, industry-funded studies proving the efficacy of fluoridated water changed the minds of dentists and public health officials. No testing of fluoride as an additive had been conducted regarding its potential health effects and fluoride had never been approved by the FDA for human ingestion.[8] Yet the fluoridation of our nation's water supplies continued. It wasn't until the 1980s that any such tests were performed. The results showed that "young male rats exposed to fluoridated water developed both bone cancer and liver cancer."[9] In the 1990s, other studies found that laboratory animals exposed to fluoridated water had Alzheimer's-like symptoms as traces of aluminum were carried to their brains. Additional studies showed an increased risk of hip fractures, motor-skills dysfunction, learning disabilities, lowered IQ levels, behavioral issues, thyroid abnormalities, arthritis, chronic fatigue syndrome, fibromyalgia and Down syndrome.

The nail in the coffin for me, regarding fluoride in the water, came from the fact that studies showed no difference in cavity rates between populations with fluoride in the water and populations without it. In fact, 17 out of 21 Western European countries have either refused or are phasing out fluoridation due to safety concerns and they have no more problems with dental decay than residents of the U.S. with fluoridated water. Direct application of fluoride using toothpaste is far more effective with fewer potential health problems. The idea that we need fluoride in the water to make up for differences in wealth or application, over time, has just not proven to be true.[10]

Chlorine: It's not just for breakfast

Safe drinking water should be a primary concern for local governments and not one that is taken lightly. Water's potential to harbor of all manner of bacterial and viral contaminants strikes fear into the hearts of men and women. At least, it should. We rarely have outbreaks of waterborne bacterial epidemics in this country and cholera outbreaks are unheard of in the U.S. That's because our water treatment plants treat our water in a number of ways, most commonly with chlorine, to prevent waterborne illnesses.[11] Unfortunately, chlorine has a number of nasty issues in and of itself.

Chlorine is an element that can transform other chemicals into mimics of estrogen, most commonly known as the female hormone. Women who drink chlorinated water are at a higher risk of developing breast cancer because chlorine reacts with some of the substances in water to form compounds that are linked to breast cancer.[12] These by-products, called trihalomethanes (THMs), are not only toxic but also carcinogenic, and have been found to be responsible for neural tube defects in babies as well as bladder and colorectal cancer in adults.[13] The most famous of the THMs is chloroform, which is why it was listed as a required test of our drinking water by the EPA. Fortunately, chloroform didn't show up in the city water tests in my area, but it is definitely there. On most days, you can smell it.

Another issue with chlorine is that, when you use hot water, whether through taking a shower or using the dishwasher, trace amounts of chlorine and other chemicals are released into the air and then inhaled and absorbed by your body. The only way to avoid this process (called "stripping") is by removing the chlorine from your water or wearing a gas mask.[14] Although I hadn't initially planned on getting a shower filter, I bought one after our water started smelling more and more like chlorine. According to Dr. Lance Wallace from the EPA, "showering is suspected as the primary cause of elevated chloroform in nearly every home because of the chlorine in the water. Chloroform levels increase up to 100 times during a ten-minute shower in residential water." This was enough to convince me to get a filter. And, after a little bit of research, I ended up buying an Aquasana shower-head filter.

Other junk

In addition to the contaminants that *do* get tested for in our water, there are a number of other potential contaminants in the water that don't get tested for, including Teflon, perchlorate and pharmaceutical and personal care product pollutants (PPCPs). Teflon in the tap water is why about 90% of us have Teflon in our blood. In higher concentrations this can lead to birth defects and development problems. Perchlorate is a rocket-fuel chemical that is also used in fireworks, flares and car airbags, and is one of those persistent chemicals that build up not only in the environment, but in your body as well. Perchlorate can cause cancer and disrupt the thyroid gland which, in turn, can negatively affect a pregnancy, resulting in mental retardation and, later, impaired motor skills for the child.[15]

Other PPCPs like birth control pills, mood stabilizers, steroids, antibiotics and pesticides can be found in increasing levels in water quality testing, yet the wastewater treatment plants aren't engineered to remove these contaminants and, as a result, they end up in our drinking water. Pharmaceuticals get into our drinking water not just from people flushing unused prescriptions down the toilet, but also from users excreting drugs in their urine. This is quite common in women who take birth control pills. No amount of chlorine treatment can eliminate these trace contaminants so, even though I don't take any of the drugs, I get a little bit every time I drink my tap water. And, of course, fish are ingesting these contaminants.

My husband came home from the Seattle Cancer Care Alliance (where he gets his cancer treatment) during this project with a brochure on the proper disposal of prescription drugs. It was pertinent not just because I was researching water quality and the junk in our water, but also because we have innumerable prescription drugs from my husband's various cancer treatments and stem cell transplants to dispose of.

The brochure listed two recommended methods for the disposal of prescription drugs. I was somewhat amused by their first suggestion, which was the preferred method. The idea was to mix unused prescription drugs with an undesirable substance (such as used coffee grounds or used kitty litter), put them in a Ziploc bag and throw them away. This method was really to prevent children and pets (and possibly dumpster divers?) from snacking on the drugs. I questioned how effective the used kitty litter and pills method would be for pet dogs since I suspect they would have regarded it as quite a tasty snack.

In any case, the brochure specifically said not to flush them down the toilet because of the danger of the drug compounds ending up in the waterways which would affect aquatic life and bring the drugs back into our drinking water. The runner-up method was to take the unused drugs to a pharmaceutical take-back location, but they strongly encouraged the first option in the federal guidelines.[16] I didn't know what they did with the drugs at the take-back locations, but I assumed they weren't flushing them down the toilet. Unfortunately, you couldn't return narcotics or controlled substances to the pharmacies on the list. Those types of drugs had to be returned to a law enforcement agency. I guess they didn't trust the employees of the take-back pharmacies to manage my huge bag of high-street-valued narcotics from when my husband was really ill.

On a side note, I didn't know what hazards there were from the degradation of the plastic-entombed pills 'n' poop combo in the landfill and the resulting goop that would leach out into the groundwater. But I suppose at the very least it was a less direct route than merely flushing them down the toilet where they could end up readily in the waterways and right back in our tap water.

Filth filter

In order to reduce or, hopefully, eliminate the fluoride, chlorine and other junk from my drinking water, a fairly sophisticated water filter was in order, one that was fine-grained enough to remove those chemicals. For that purpose, I looked into a carbon water filter. Other types of filtration waste a lot of water in the process (like alkaline water machines) or are extremely expensive to implement (whole house or reverse osmosis systems). For the purposes of this project and the future, I wanted to stick with something that was easy to obtain, install and use and that wasn't going to cost an arm and a leg.

In searching for a water filter to not only remove some of the additives and contaminants in our water but also improve the palatability (no more eau de bleach et algae!), I was concerned about investing in a whole house system, since our water was relatively decent to start with. Even though I wanted to get a carbon-filtering pitcher-type contraption, I was worried about BPA, phthalates and other plasticizers in the container since they all, inevitably, are made out of plastic. I had yet to see a stainless steel or glass filtration system.

After doing a bit of research, I managed to find the EcoFlo Family Water Pitcher which was free from BPA, PVC and phthalates.[17] Another nice benefit of this filter was that you could use it with any type of water source either from the tap or from rainwater, rivers, streams or even lakes. I know this sounds a little like end-of-civilization extremism, but I took comfort in knowing that, if there was ever an issue with our water supply, I could filter rainwater, water from our rain barrel (that stores clean, captured house water for our vegetable plants) or stream water in an emergency. It just didn't do salt water, so I would need to stay out of Puget Sound for my drinking water needs.

This pitcher removed up to 99.99% of contaminants found in drinking water and it filtered fast, unlike other pitcher filters I had used 10 years ago when we were living in California and the drinking water was unpalatable. The EcoFlo filtered DDT, PCBs, detergents, pesticides, chlorine, aluminum, asbestos, cadmium, chromium 6, benzene, copper, lead, arsenic and mercury, and microscopic pathogens such as cryptosporidium, giardia, cholera, E. coli, salmonella and anthrax, of all things. It actually filtered out quite a bit more than the ones listed, but those are the more noteworthy ones. As for the fluoride, it didn't remove all of it, just about 65%.

Clearing the air

Just as we started this project, our vacuum cleaner of 20 years finally presented itself beyond repair. In other words, it kicked the bucket. I much prefer trying to fix something rather than throwing it out and buying a new one. Since this was a nice canister vacuum and replacing it would be expensive, we had opted in the past to get it repaired. A few years ago the motor on the carpet attachment burned out because I decided to vacuum our flokati rug one too many times. And then the main motor burned out, so we took the whole thing in for repair, which was more difficult than it sounded.

Our dead vacuum was a Kenmore and apparently it was not legal for most vacuum repair shops to work on Kenmore vacuums—it had to be taken to a special Sears repair shop. There weren't too many of these shops in our area and trying to schedule and arrange a weekday drop-off and pick-up was a pain but, for less than the price of a new one, we got it fixed and got a few more years out of it. Then the vacuum hose started falling apart and popping out frequently. When the vacuum cleaner wasn't popping out the hose, it was dropping pieces that held the electrical cord in it. In any case, it was time to replace it.

Fortunately, replacing our vacuum was high on my list of things to do for this project because I wanted to get a true HEPA (High Efficiency Particulate Air) sealed-system vacuum. It all sounds very technical but basically I was looking for a vacuum with a HEPA filter that filtered particulates as small as .3 microns and that was housed in a sealed system so that the particulates vacuumed up couldn't escape out the back end. This is potentially a problem in nonsealed system vacuums. I didn't want to spend the money on a purportedly HEPA vacuum only to find out that it just picked up big chunks and then shot the smaller bits right back out again.

The reason for having an extremely effective vacuum and, of course, using it frequently, is that most household dust contains a whole lot of lead, PFOS (Scotchgard and the like) and PBDEs (flame retardants). These are the most common contaminants of concern. The lead comes from paint chipping, carpeting and dirt carried in from outside. The PFOS comes from stain-resistant coating on carpeting and furniture. PBDEs come from electronic dust from computers, televisions, monitors and the like and the flame retardants that poof out from your furniture every time you sit down on something that contains foam. So, unless you have only wood chairs and nonpadded church pews to sit on, it is in pretty much everything else. And, since this project didn't include our replacing all of our padded furniture, it was important to address this issue using a different route.

The big problem wasn't so much just replacing our canister vacuum with a true HEPA, sealed-system one, it was finding one that fit this criteria and didn't cost an arm and a leg. I didn't want to spend a thousand dollars on a vacuum. Most of the vacuums available at that price range seemed to be gimmicks that broke down just as quickly as the cheaper ones. I wanted a vacuum that would last, so I was willing to pay more than a few hundred dollars. After hours spent researching allergy and healthy home product websites and reading dozens of reviews, I settled on a low- to mid-range Miele.

Our new vacuum was a product from a manufacturer that allegedly took into account long-lasting product lines since they still made available parts for vacuums that were sold over a decade ago. Most manufacturers of appliances employ the business tactic of planned obsolescence so you are forced into purchasing a new product when the old one wears out either because you can't find anyone who knows how to fix it or because replacement parts don't exist anymore. This has become a bigger issue with single molded-plastic pieces in everything from vacuums to refrigerators. For the most part it has become cheaper to replace the whole appliance rather than fix the problem. We had a similar issue with our relatively new GE Profile refrigerator when a plastic door-seal part snapped off. It would have cost us $800 to "fix" it, which was really just replacing the door as there was no other way of attaching it back to the rest of the door. Miele, on the other hand, had a history of solid construction and replacement parts, so I felt less buyer's remorse investing $500 in a vacuum.

In any case, this lightweight, quiet vacuum was an immense improvement over our old vacuum that no doubt put back just as much dust into the air as it was picking up. I sprung for the upgraded HEPA filter on our new vacuum just to ensure that, when we vacuumed, we were picking up all those flame-retardant and lead bits and pieces and keeping them in the canister rather than spraying them right back into my sinuses. Since I ordered it through Amazon, we got the vacuum about a day later and I went to town testing it out, not only for its ability to pick up all the dirt and crud the kids tend to drag into the house (really, "Take your shoes off!" and "Turn off the water!" should be engraved on my eco-friendly grave marker), but also to see how much the vacuum smelled. Any new appliance is going to off-gas a little heated-up plasticky smell as the plastic, lube and grease gets exercised the first few times.

One thing that was a little alarming about the vacuum was that the "exhaust," rather than coming out the back of the canister like it did in our old vacuum, shot straight up into the air, like a geyser. I really hated the back-end exhaust action, because all it did was shoot fuzz balls, dirt and dust bunnies back into an area you had already vacuumed if you had it aimed the wrong direction. However, the geyser method, although unnerving when you accidentally crossed your head into its jet stream and got blown all over the place (well, my hair that is), avoided the dirt redistribution method employed by the other one.

The geyser method also allowed you to smell, or rather, not smell, the exhaust. Our old vacuum had a stink about it. Not just dirty air flying out the back end, but also something like a burning dirt mixed with a chemical smell. You could always tell when it was recently used, just because it left a stink in the house. And it wasn't just because it was old. It always left this stink. The new Miele one, however, was like a breath of fresh air. I honestly didn't mind getting my face caught in the geyser stream because it was more like a fan blowing clean air instead of exhaust fumes.

As for its cleaning power, it was well worth the price of admission. It was extremely quiet, even with the carpet cleaning attachment affixed and it vacuumed better than any vacuum I've ever owned. I actually *wanted* to vacuum. I would go out of my way to vacuum areas of the house even if I had vacuumed them recently. Because it was lightweight, quiet and easy to maneuver, didn't smell and, most importantly, made me feel like I was sterilizing the house from a bunch of chemical dust, I was motivated to whip out the vacuum. Which, for me, was a bloody miracle.

Leafy indoor air purifying

For about a month before we got our new vacuum, my mom kept asking us whether or not we wanted a Peace Lily plant that she had received from one of her friends. It turned out that her friend from her Senior Center exercise group liked to propagate Peace Lilies and had a ton to give away. My mom was one of the lucky recipients. Unfortunately, she's not that big into houseplants. When I was growing up, the majority of plants we had in the house were of the plastic variety.

One day, not too long after these conversations, she showed up with the plant tucked away in a Styrofoam drip tray. I put it on our fireplace mantel and promptly ignored it until I had time to give it a permanent home. However, as I started researching indoor air purifiers, mostly of the HEPA variety as well as plants that help clean the air of your home, I saw that Peace Lilies were considered to be one of the best plants for purifying indoor air. I immediately took note and got that Peace Lily a brand new home and put it in a prominent place in the house.

I had already been planning on using plants for indoor air quality since I wasn't sure if I wanted to spring the money for the specialized air purifiers that address environmental chemicals. Most of the machine-based purifiers (in other words, not plants) were geared to filter out dust and allergens and weren't made to work on PDBEs, metals and the like. I was already wondering how effective an air purifier would be anyway, unless I got one specifically for chemical filtration. I also was not interested in getting an air purifier the size of an armchair and as loud as a bus. I've been around the more industrial air purifiers and, while they do the job, they are big and annoying.

On the other hand, we are really lackadaisical about houseplants. At the time, we only had two plants in the house and both were of the low-maintenance cactus variety. When my husband underwent his stem cell transplants, we were instructed to remove all cut flowers and house plants during that year because of the risk of infection from bacteria in the flowers and from mold in the dirt. Even though his immune system was mostly recovered (he was still on a number of immune suppressants), we had not gone out of our way to get any new plants. The only reason we had two cacti was because my kids went through a period of absolute fixation with anything related to deserts. Since we couldn't move to the desert, we brought a little bit of desert to us.

In any case, if we were going to turn our home into a lush tropical oasis for cleaning the air, we needed plants that were easy to care for and required minimal maintenance. So I was happy to read that our Peace Lily, aka Spathiphyllum, didn't need much in the way of excessive light or water to survive. More importantly, it cleaned indoor air of many environmental contaminants including benzene, formaldehyde, trichloroethylene and other pollutants like toluene and xylene. Back in the 1980s, NASA reported some research it did on the value of indoor plants in cleaning up air quality. There was a lot of concern over the hazardous working environment in Skylab, given the fact that the synthetic materials inside emitted more than 100 chemicals. What made a good air-cleaning plant had more to do with the type of bacteria that the plant encouraged around its roots and in its leaves since it's those micro-organisms that break down the chemicals. Over the years, researchers have looked at more than 30 different plants to find the ones that are best at cleaning indoor air.[18]

Not wanting to just stuff the house full of one kind of plant, even though the Peace Lily was allegedly one of the "best" plants for the job, I went in search of some other plants to liven things up. To purify the indoor air of your home, you need 15 to 20 houseplants for a 1,800 square foot home.[19] Since we spent most of our time on the main floor and little in the basement, I focused on just that part of the house. I figured about 15 houseplants (from the recommended list) would do the job nicely.

Other research done over the years has shown that many indoor plants reduce volatile organic compounds by up to 100% over 24 hours in a closed environment. In fact, a spider plant alone can remove 80% of formaldehyde pollutants from an enclosed room in 24 hours.[20] What was even more important, since we lived in Seattle (the land of mold and mildew), was that these plants cleaned the air by metabolizing pollutants drawn in through their leaves and emitted a substance that suppressed the growth of mold, spores and bacteria.[21]

Since we had an enormous mold problem in our master bathroom and, as a result, our bedroom (we didn't have a fan in the attached bathroom), the first places I targeted for plants were the bedroom and bathroom in addition to the living room. I didn't mind having plants that not only cleaned the air of chemical contaminants, but also helped deal with our mold and mildew issues which were nearly impossible to control without some toxic chemicals themselves (about which I'll go into further detail later).

On my shortlist of plants to buy was a spider plant (which battles benzene, formaldehyde, carbon monoxide and xylene), a gerbera daisy for the dining room (trichloroethylene and benzene), snake plant for the bathroom (formaldehyde), dracaena for the bedroom (xylene, trichloroethylene and formaldehyde), aloe vera for the kitchen (formaldehyde and benzene) and English ivy for the kids' bathroom (reduces airborne fecal matter).[22] I had recently moved a dwarf banana plant indoors since it didn't like being outside during the fall or winter in our area. Since it was a tropical plant, I thought I'd look into its air-purifying possibilities, even though I hadn't yet seen it on the other plant lists. Lo and behold, I found it on the shortlist in an article on the Daily Green website.[23] That list led me to another list which had on it, prominently, a Christmas cactus (not actually a cactus), which I had also recently purchased.[24]

One last thing I found out about house plants was that those planted in plastic pots or grown in a nursery where a lot of pesticides were used can off-gas more volatile organic compounds (VOCs) than previously thought.[25] As I found plants for the house, I made sure to repot them into nonplastic containers. The afternoon I purchased six houseplants to get our air purifying project under way, I immediately noticed a difference in the air quality in our bedroom. However, I think it was all psychological that after a few hours in the room two plants could have made that much difference.

Emma got a *Dieffenbachia camilla* for her bedroom (aka Dumb Cane), which she named Cammy. Of course, it's the only potentially toxic plant that I bought so I needed to make sure she didn't start nibbling on it. Plus, the sap it produced can be a skin irritant, so if she started playing with it, I would relocate it somewhere safer. Emma spent the afternoon sitting in front of it, talking to it and having her toy animals play on it. Needless to say, she was a happy customer. The plant, on the other hand, didn't like her room so much, either from the shady corner I put it in or because of the temperature. I ended up having to move it to the living room.

Henry, on the other hand, for some weird reason started to freak out about all the new houseplants. I know it's not unusual for him to be resistant to change but I didn't think he would have such a severe meltdown about it — it ended with him lying on my bed and kicking his feet, screaming, "No more plants!" Apparently, everywhere he looked he claimed he could see a new plant. And I still wasn't anywhere near the recommended 15 to 20 houseplants. I even suggested any new ones go downstairs, until he got used to them, but that just elicited even more tantrums. Even an ornamental pepper got him all riled up.

I still really didn't understand what the aversion to the plants was, but he got used to the ones I bought and over the following months I managed to sneak in a few more when he wasn't paying attention. Which was pretty much never. But a plant here and a plant there brought us up to 16 plants before he had another fit of, "No more plants! I hate plants! They bother me! Everywhere I look there's a plant!" Henry only likes cactus plants, and if you bring home anything else it's a problem.

Emma's birthday bash

My daughter's birthday is right before Halloween and each year we have a small birthday party where she can invite over her friends for whatever activity she's interested in with cake and presents. The previous year she wanted some arts and crafts project as the main activity and this year was no different. That made it relatively easy, since she wanted to decorate t-shirts with fabric pens. We already had a stack of non-toxic fabric pens that are always a hit, and I picked up some t-shirts for her and her friends to decorate. Initially, Emma had wanted the t-shirts that were like coloring book pages (she has one of them), but when I went to the store, they didn't have any in their sizes so I opted for plain pink and yellow shirts.

In order to spice things up a little bit, I also bought a variety of iron-on fabric decorations for them to design their own shirts and then decorate with the fabric pens. I spent far too much time in the aisles of the store attempting to suss out what potential toxins I was going to expose them to. Anything heated up with an iron is suspect for airborne toxins and I immediately decided that the rhinestone iron-on decorations were potentially a problem given the fact that they were manufactured in China and most likely had some lead content. I did end up picking up a few small crystal (most likely glass) iron-ons since the metal content looked negligible and really the only thing of concern was the adhesive.

For people who do a lot of crafting with rhinestones, you can affix them using rhinestone adhesive glue. The big issue with the tube of glue (versus the iron-on adhesive) is that it contains perchloroethylene, which is a known carcinogen. This is the same chemical that is used in dry-cleaning clothes and can cause a number of health issues. Long-term exposure can cause damage to the central nervous system and can cause leukemia and cancer of the skin, colon, lung, larynx, bladder and urogenital tract. Not something you want to get for your birthday.

The more I looked into rhinestone adhesive tape as well as iron-on adhesive, the less I could determine what the heck they were actually made of. It's amazing how so much marketing and advertising goes into a product, but so little of what the actual product materials are is mentioned. This makes perfect sense to some degree because most people don't care and wouldn't know what to do with the information anyway. When you throw in the issue of product formulation secrecy it's almost impossible to find out what's in something as simple, yet so chemically complicated, as iron-on transfers. The safest thing would be to opt for something where I knew exactly what I was dealing with, but I also didn't want to completely drop the project. Most of the other art project ideas I had for her birthday party all involved toxins in some form or other — most craft paints have toxic colorants and it's the same story with toxins in clay.

It was getting down to the wire, with two days before Emma's party, and I needed to make a decision. After spending far too much time researching, I finally discovered — after contacting a company that manufactured the iron-on adhesives — that the fabric appliqués used a non-toxic adhesive. It was the same story with the glass iron-ons, so we ended up using those for her t-shirt coloring birthday party after all. When I was ironing them on during the party, I could smell some chemical-type smells, but nothing too overwhelming. I was worried but, at that point, it was too late anyway. I wasn't going to tell a group of hopped-up six-year-olds to give me back the appliqués they had so carefully designed.

My husband was, again, in charge of the birthday cake. He was working on some new recipes and since I was sick the weekend of the party, I really wasn't paying too close attention to what he was doing with the cake. It wasn't until I went into the kitchen after cleaning the bathroom that I noticed he had the cake covered in pink frosting and was working on some green frosting for decorating. I hadn't been thinking of the food coloring issue again with the cake, but if it was any consolation, the amount was negligible compared to the coal tar cake, aka Red Velvet, that we had had for my husband's birthday a few weeks earlier. I reminded myself that I really needed to get on with ordering the natural food coloring kit for my husband to try out before it got too close to another birthday.

Treats for the party consisted of all-organic apples, carrots and crackers. Emma's family birthday dinner, which followed the party with her friends, was made up of a lot of organic items from our sailboat community supported agriculture (CSA). For the tail end of the summer we were getting a farm share from a sailboat-delivered CSA program. It's not a true CSA in that you don't pay money up front to buy the season's produce and you can opt in and out depending on your schedule and inclinations, but all the produce we got was local, organic, in season and transported in a carbon-neutral way from farm to dock to pick-up site.

The produce was shipped via sailboat, and transported to the pick-up location by electric truck. The program is run through the Salish Sea Trading Cooperative. I am an acquaintance of one of the co-owners, Kathy Pelish. The idea is to become more reliant on local food sources where you have not only complete knowledge of the growing methods (organic or not; use of petroleum, pesticides, fertilizers and the like), but also complete control over the amount of petroleum that went into the transportation of the produce. A lot of press has been given to the number of miles your food travels to get from farm to plate, so creating a local carbon-neutral resource for delivering and supporting local agriculture is important in reducing those miles. As someone who has worked on the local Puget Sound Fresh program for more than nine years, I'm a huge proponent of supporting local agriculture, preserving farmland and keeping farming small and sustainable. In any case, treats and the family dinner for Emma's birthday comprised many items from our CSA box that week.

The birthday treats that I brought in for her first grade class the following day, however, were an epic non-toxic fail. I had planned on making cookies, but I had a nasty chest cold and didn't have the energy to pull that off the day after her birthday party in spite of my good intentions. Instead, I went to the store and bought cookies. I could have gone to Whole Foods (aka Whole Paycheck) and gotten 30-odd cookies for God knows how much, which still would have been considerably less than the $100 it would have cost to get the local, organic cupcakes that I would have really liked to get. Or the $65 for the local, hand-forged donuts they love.

I just put my fingers in my ears and pretended that I didn't hear my brain yelling at me that I should have gotten cookies that didn't have food coloring and cookies that were organic and didn't have traces of pesticides in them and the high-fructose corn syrup that had traces of mercury in it. What I was listening to was the fact that my kids love the cookies that I did buy and that they would think it was a super-special treat since I never buy them for them and that they would be happy because of that. And that I hadn't yet really started the food portion of the project and, furthermore, I wasn't eating them now was I? Even so, I believe part of my avenger cape got caught in the gears that day.

Happy Birthday! Here's your bra (.) (.)

The day after Emma turned seven, I started seeing some news about the studies that had just come out showing that girls ages seven and eight were more likely today than in the past to start developing breasts. This is a problem not just from a teasing and self-esteem perspective, let alone a hormone-spiked behavioral one, but also from a health perspective. Girls who experience early puberty are at higher risk of breast and endometrial cancer as well as elevated blood pressure due to longer lifetime exposure to the hormones estrogen and progesterone.[26] While higher rates of obesity, lower birth weight and formula feeding are all thought to be possible reasons for girls developing earlier, environmental toxins have also been proposed as a possible trigger and studies are being done to test this hypothesis.

In a study reported in 2010, involving about 1,240 seven-year-old girls, 10.4% of white, 23.4% of black and 14.9% of Hispanic girls had enough breast development to be considered at the onset of puberty. At age eight, 18.3% of white, 42.9% of black and 30.9% of Hispanic girls were beginning puberty. The percentages found were much higher than those seen in a 1997 study.[27] Of the white girls in the newer study, twice as many seven-year-olds had started breast development as the girls in the study done 10 years earlier.[28] In other studies, accidental exposure to high levels of toxins, as seen among farm families in Michigan exposed to the flame retardant PBB, can be the cause of some cases of early puberty. Additionally, studies of BPA, which is a hormone disruptor, has shown that exposure during critical periods of development may cause early puberty.[29]

I remembered that the previous spring I was talking to the mom of a second grader who was starting to exhibit signs of early puberty. I really felt almost blindsided by it all. I figured I had years before I needed to have "the talk" with my daughter about not only puberty but also sex and the rest. I knew that there was a downward trend with younger girls developing earlier, but I figured it was still rare. But here I was talking to a real live mom of one of these girls. It makes sense, if more than 1 in 10 girls are exhibiting signs of early puberty at age seven, that more second graders would be on an earlier course as well. Of course, I joked about giving her daughter too much rBGH-laced milk. Hormones, or rather, hormone-disrupting contaminants (since there is no hard data linking rBGH to early puberty), are acting on young bodies in a way we don't really understand yet.

Other chemicals besides BPA (which gets the most news coverage) that potentially disrupt hormones are some preservatives, cleansers and plastic additives. According to Ted Schettler, MD, MPH, Science Director for the Science and Environmental Health Network, "young girls are exposed to dozens of potentially toxic chemicals on a daily basis. Some of these can mimic the natural hormone, estrogen. Although individually their estrogenic activity may be relatively weak, their effects are additive. In the aggregate they could be having significant health effects, including contributing to the early onset of breast development."[30]

While Emma wasn't showing early signs of puberty, and I hoped it stayed that way for a while, I certainly didn't think it was worth the risk of exposure if we still don't know what these hormone disruptors do to growing girls. And boys, for that matter. Clearly, part of this project was to eliminate most of the contaminants like BPA, phthalates, parabens and the like and for that, I was re-energized about taking on the role of the Non-toxic Avenger in our household, just to help protect my family. I did understand, of course, that there might be no link between these chemicals and the trends we were seeing but, as far as I was concerned and given the other health issues around our house, why take the chance when there are alternatives available that completely eliminate that potential risk?

Halloween

I love Halloween. It's one of my favorite holidays. I can't say this has always been the case as I never was big into the adult parties or wearing costumes or even decorating. It wasn't until I had kids that Halloween was even on my radar. When Henry was five months old we were invited to a neighbor's house for an infant Halloween party. I can honestly claim that the last Halloween party I had been to up until then was when I was in elementary school.

Hank and I were always conscientious about making sure we had enough treats for the neighborhood children but, when we had kids, we became a lot more aware of what people were handing out. When the kids were very young we would take them trick-or-treating but, inevitably, one of them would get scared a few houses into it and we'd end up back at home. This wasn't that much of an issue since it gave them a chance to get a little candy but not so much that we'd have to deal with Halloween candy into January. This is still pretty much the case. Henry has a little more stamina than Emma, but we still aren't out for very long, which I honestly don't mind at all.

More importantly, our kids have a lot more fun answering the door at home and handing out treats than actually going out and getting it themselves. Even when Henry was only two and a half, he was intrigued by handing out candy. That year, we had pretty much closed up shop for the evening and turned out the lights because it was late and the kids needed to get to bed. I was giving Emma a bath (she was only a year old at the time) and my husband was downstairs doing laundry. I didn't hear the doorbell ringing since the bath water was running. It wasn't until I heard the door close that I realized that some older kids had come to the house trick-or-treating and Henry had answered the door and handed out candy. I'm sure the kids who came to the door thought it was odd that a two-year-old was handing out candy without an adult in sight.

The trend of Henry and Emma handing out candy hasn't changed much except that nowadays I prescreen who will be answering the door based on what's waiting on the other side. One year Henry opened the door, with me standing behind it, so I couldn't really see who was on the other side. He dropped the candy bowl and disappeared in a flash. He wasn't too thrilled with the creepy costumed ax-murdering teenager who greeted him.

Every year I have to make some tough decisions about what we get for not just Halloween costumes, but for candy and decorations because so much of it is made out of some really nasty materials. The best-looking decorations usually contain the worst-smelling stuff. A lot of the window clings and bloody, drippy hands and body parts are made out of vinyl, PVC or some unidentifiable, greasy, phthalate-filled plastic material. This year, since we were doing this project, it was even more difficult. We had some plastic decorations which were most likely safe but, since they went outside anyway, we wouldn't be breathing anything in on the off-chance they decided to off-gas. Some of our decorations were made of wood and metal and I think the fake cobwebs were safe. The ceramic, plastic, paper and cardboard decorations were fine, but all the vinyl window clings and other gory stuff stayed in the storage boxes.

A big issue was with the kids' costumes. We had never done the rubber or vinyl masks, mostly because of the high stink factor. This year they were certainly a big no-no because of the plasticizers and potential phthalates in them. The masks sit right on the face and I didn't want my kids breathing that stuff in for any length of time. Hard plastic masks were most likely okay, but Henry and Emma generally don't choose costumes that have masks. I looked into our face paints and they were all non-toxic paints, so if they wanted anything on their faces, it would be face paints. Face paints can contain lead, nickel, cobalt and chromium, depending on the color, so you have to be careful with them.[31] I tried to stick to more natural fabrics or come up with a costume that wasn't pre-packaged, although my kids were pretty picky about them. The worst thing was the potential for fabrics that contained flame retardants.

This year, we wouldn't be burning any candles made out of paraffin. Usually I would get rid of some old petroleum-based emergency tea candles in the pumpkins outside, but this year I planned on burning soy candles. I couldn't bring myself to waste beeswax candles in the pumpkins since they are so much more expensive, I love the smell of them and I couldn't imagine burning them without enjoying it myself. In any case, all the candles would be non-toxic, even the ones outside.

Halloween candies were already all over the stores and I couldn't help but think about the nonstick packaging in all those candy wrappers. I never really knew what made those candy wrappers so slippery on the inside so that the sometimes melted chocolate and gooey caramel inside didn't stick like glue. My mom has a habit of providing us with bags of candy for handing out at Halloween because she can get them on sale, not too dissimilar from the school supplies thing. This time I needed to make sure I warned her ahead of time not to get us anything as I had planned on making our treat handouts as toxin-free as possible.

We live in a development in Seattle that is known for trick-or-treating, so parents will drive their kids out here for a night of fun. Since we are one of the few neighborhoods in North Seattle with sidewalks and tucked away from traffic, we get a lot of kids. We can easily go through 10 bags of candy before we have to turn off the lights and let people know we are done for the evening. The last few years I started adding in non-candy items to our Halloween candy bowl, mostly pencils and other little toys. This year I planned to make sure that all of our candy was the kind wrapped in foil or cellophane with a mix of non-toxic pencils and erasers and the like.

Pfucked by PFCs

Shortly before Halloween, I received an email from a colleague letting me know they were doing a Halloween blog post round-up and asking if I had any suggestions. I hadn't yet posted my screed on PVCs and PFCs (perfluorinated compounds found in Teflon and stain-resistant products) in Halloween decorations, costumes and candy all in relation to the research I was doing for this book. Sarah, from the blog *Practically Green*, asked a bit more about the book and, of course, in the process I went to look something up to back up a statement I had made about PFCs. That's when I stumbled upon The List.[32] Someone had put together a fairly comprehensive list of items (both household and other) that had some sort of perfluorinated compound involved in their manufacture.

As I read through The List I realized that getting rid of perfluorinated compounds was going to be a lot harder than it sounded. My laptop cord had recently started flaking out on me and I ended up using electrical tape to hold the wiring together while I waited for the new power cord to ship out. I glanced down at that electrical tape as soon as I saw it on The List and gave it a dirty look. I was also pretty sure my laptop cord had some sort of PFC coating on it as well since it has that sort of shiny, greasy look to it. In addition, wire insulation was on the list so I didn't doubt it was coating my laptop as well.

A lot of the stuff on the list I already knew about and we were slowly reducing and eliminating its usage, most of it in the kitchen. The plastic kitchen utensils (mostly spatulas), nonstick pans and clothing were high on my list of items that were purged. But then there was my hair dryer, my flat iron, the clothes iron and the ironing board cover. All nonstick coating. Anything smacking of stain resistance, waterproofing and water repellant was suspect, but what about some of the other things I found?

Dental floss? Pfuck. We had tried switching over to a more natural brand in the past, mostly to reduce our plastic usage. Eco-Dent, the natural brand, came in cardboard packaging, but didn't work as well as the Reach waxed dental floss we had been using forever. And because Reach works better we stuck with it. There are no ingredient listings on our Reach dental floss and I couldn't find any information on the Johnson & Johnson website. However, after poking around a bit more, I did discover that anything with "easy glide" or "Gore" and some tape-styles of dental floss were made out of PTFEs (a type of PFC). Colgate Total, Oral-B Satin Floss, Butler GUM Eez-Thru, Reach Easy Slide and Crest Glide were made out of Teflon or PTFE, but I still didn't know about our regular Reach floss. Even though I suspected it was made from nylon we still switched to Eco-Dent. And then switched back again. We still didn't like it.

When I went hunting through our cabinets looking for other dental floss and their potential PTFE contaminants, I noticed we also had a package of DenTek Complete Clean that we had used on occasion—but only when we ran out of our other floss. We both hated it because it was like flossing with piano wire. It was torture on the gums and made them bleed. My husband who, because of chemo, has more sensitive gums and dental needs suffered especially. Upon closer inspection, the floss just looked like two strands of woven nylon but when I checked their website those two strands were two strands of PTFE floss.[33] It went into the giveaway pile.

What about denture cleansers? Pfucked again. My husband used Efferdent to clean his night guard and I occasionally used it as well. It did a bang-up job of cleaning the lumps of plastic that were soaking in spittle all night long, being ground into oblivion. What's the ingredient list, you ask? Among a few other questionable things, polytetrafluoroethylene (our friend PTFE) was listed as a "processing aid." I wondered what, exactly, it was processing. We managed to find a different product, Polident, that didn't have PTFE in it. At least, it wasn't listed.

Rounding out the list were things we just didn't have much control over. Prescription containers, which my husband went through a lot of every month, weren't exactly negotiable. The pharmacists weren't going to switch over to a different material and, really, since I was the one trying to follow this project more closely for testing purposes, and since I didn't take any medication, this one issue was moot.

Why so much pfear over PFCs? PFOA, which is a breakdown product of PFCs, does not degrade. At all. It has a half-life in humans of more than four years and, since we are continually renewing our exposure through things like dental floss in our mouths and stain-resistant clothing on our skin, it is something to think about. Studies have shown that PFOAs can damage the liver as well as other organs. They can cause immune and endocrine disruption. In 2006, the EPA upgraded PFOA to a "likely human carcinogen" in response to evidence that it can cause testicular, pancreatic, mammary and liver tumors. It was described as an "indestructible toxic chemical group that pollutes nearly every American's blood."[34]

Not-so-sweet dreams

I used to sleep on my stomach. I absolutely loved sleeping on my stomach. My husband used to make fun of me because I would tuck my hands under my legs and he said I looked like some sort of turbo sleeper. In fact, I believe he even called it the "turbo position." Because of the strain this position put on my neck I had, over the years, learned to tuck some old stuffed critter under one of my shoulders to raise it a little. It sounds weird now, that I was still sleeping with a stuffed animal, but it was really only a convenient sleeping device not unlike a body pillow or some other strategically placed sleep aid. So, I had to guard that squished stuffed Pink Panther that my husband won at a carnival game in Vegas from our dog like my life depended on it. Nobody messed with Pink Panther. And he came with us whenever we travelled.

About 10 years earlier I had really started having neck and upper back pain, mostly due to sitting at the computer for hours on end, programming at work, but I had also strained the muscles from over-exercising my tight muscles. After a particularly bad bout of back pain I went to the doctor who referred me to a specialist and the first thing he told me to do was to stop sleeping on my stomach. I couldn't imagine a more annoying prescription. How do you change the way you've been sleeping for almost 30 years? Pink Panther was relegated to the closet to be covered in dust bunnies and eventually go to those pink clouds in the sky.

I wasn't looking forward to not-so-restful sleep but the alternative was worse. Pain trumps tiredness every time. I persevered with other sleeping positions and ended up looking for a new bed pillow to help out with sleeping on my side. Sleeping on my back was unimaginable but side sleeping was at least doable. At the time, I worked not too far away from a Relax The Back store so I sauntered in one day (more like stiffly ambled—I still couldn't really turn my head) looking for help. One of the salespeople suggested a Tempur-Pedic contoured neck pillow. She had me lie down on one of the beds to test out the correct size of pillow as I lay on my side.

After this somewhat uncomfortable demonstration I gingerly got up and emptied my wallet to pay for it. Spending $125 or so on a pillow seemed out of control since I think the most I had paid in the past was $20, but maybe that was the source of my problem. And I was certainly sold on the whole "developed by physicians to promote proper support" and "relieves shoulder, neck and back pain by allowing the neck and shoulder muscles to relax completely." It sounded exactly like what I needed. Except that it weighed a ton. It smelled like a chemical factory. And you could only sleep on one quarter of the pillow because of the contouring. You couldn't flip it over and use the other side. You had to make sure it was always placed properly—no fluffing and throwing yourself down on the pillow. Even if you did, it would feel like you're hitting cement. Did I mention it weighed a ton?

But I loved it, stinky warts and all. Because of its enormous heft, I could never take it traveling and I always missed it terribly when out of town. Most hotel pillows were overstuffed or lumpy or just plain impossible to sleep on. I would kick myself for not bringing it along and my husband would mention the same old story about how President Bush always traveled with his pillow. But President Bush was a pussy—nobody traveled with their pillow except little kids, right? Especially if your pillow weighed more than your luggage.

As I started examining the chemical flame retardants in mattresses and children's sleepwear, I started to think about what else we were sleeping on. I hadn't really given my pillow much thought but I knew, because of its age, that I should look into replacing it. Tempur-Pedic claims that its material is resistant to dust mites and whatnot, but knowing that feather and synthetic pillows are a "cesspool of mold, mildew, fungus, dust mites and mite feces," according to bedding expert Dan Schecter, I couldn't imagine that 10 years of sweat, skin cells and dust weren't working some sort of magic in my Tempur-Pedic as well.[35]

My kids, who now also sleep on their stomachs and will hopefully not face the same fate as I have, always made fun of my brick-like pillow. They never understood why it weighed a ton and forever asked why I slept on such a strange thing. Tempur-Pedic material is strange indeed, and the company guards the formula for it closely, with only a handful of individuals at Tempur-Pedic made privy to the proprietary trade secret ingredients. The actual materials that go into making the layers of this high-density polyurethane memory foam is unknown, but some websites have suggested that it is a petroleum-based product with the potential for off-gassing a number of contaminants including acetaldehyde, benzene, limonene, toluene and styrene.[36]

Getting back to their dust- and allergen-free claim, every Tempur-Pedic product is "sprayed with an anti-allergen treatment designed to prevent dust, mold and mites from infesting or getting inside the mattress."[37] I hate to think what that spray consists of, but hopefully not some modern day DDT. And, just like mattresses, most memory foam contains a flame retardant, which is even more important since, based on what I found, it sounded like the Tempur-Pedic material was even more flammable than the average pillow. Since it uses body heat to accomplish its "memory" action, too much heat can cause it to melt.[38] That's a whole lot of chemicals to be breathing in every night, along with the dust mites, mold, fungus and all.

A considerable number of people have complained of health issues after sleeping on a Tempur-Pedic bed or pillow. Most are related to allergic reactions but other claims include headache, nausea, pain, disturbing dreams and other issues that haven't exactly been corroborated so it's all anecdotal at this point. But, given the materials and the high level of stink and off-gassing, it's certainly not impossible that there are some effects going on. In any case, I needed a new pillow and I wasn't about to replace it with something even potentially toxic so I started researching my healthy and natural pillow options.

I wasn't really interested in a noisy or hard pillow, like something made out of buckwheat hulls. Nor did I want something that I knew would compress over time, like organic cotton. I've slept on one too many futons in my lifetime and I know what sort of leaden lump those turn into, regardless of how much fluffing and turning you do to them. The other options were kapok seeds, 100% wool or natural latex. The latex reminded me too much of the memory foam, but it was an option I was willing to look into. I wasn't sure about the kapok. I was really interested in the all-wool pillow, but since you can't wash it I didn't want to have it around all the people in my house who tend to barf. A lot. I decided to go with a nonallergenic down pillow. We already had several goose down comforters and, although I've read that down tends to attract more dust mites and mold, washing it several times a year and having a cover on it helps keep that problem down.

I found an eco-friendly, allergy-free down pillow with an organic cotton cover that fit the bill. It was expensive, but I didn't want to spring for a cheap one that would lump up over time, or that didn't meet my requirements for being non-toxic and nonallergenic. I also bought an organic cotton case for the pillow to keep out moisture and dust mites to further protect my investment. I was really concerned that it wouldn't work as well as my Tempur-Pedic pillow and that I'd have to work my way through several different kinds of pillows before I found the right one.

Since it's hard to find natural pillows in bedding stores, you can't really experience what they feel like until you've bought them online and by then it's too late. Pillows are like underwear and bathing suits—once you've taken them out of the package and tried them out for a while you can't return them. I guess they don't want to restock a pillow full of drool. In any case, if the down pillow I ordered ended up not being comfortable, my husband would get it as a replacement since he needed a new one and I would try the wool. And we would just try to keep the barfers away from it. However, I ended up liking my down pillow so much I didn't need to look any further.

Getting down

As I mentioned before, we had a down comforter that we used on our bed. Up until this project, our kids had used a variety of blankets that were an odd mishmash of crocheted blankets handmade by my grandmother, polyester blankets given as presents or purchased and a mix of fleece blankets that I "made" by just buying fleece fabric from the fabric store. We all loved the fleece blankets. They came in a huge variety of bright patterns, like the pirate skeletons and the solar system ones that my son used, the flowered ones my daughter used and the cowgirl one I used as a throw on the couch.

The big problem with the fleece blankets, aside from the fact that they were made from petroleum, was that they were highly flammable. The fabric I purchased to make these blankets and throws wasn't treated with PDBEs, which is fine by me, but if there was a fire, the fleece would melt like plastic wrap onto our sleeping bodies. Which freaked the hell out of me. Once I realized this lovely tidbit while researching flame retardants, bedding and sleepwear, I immediately went on a quest to replace the fleece blankets on the beds with natural bedding materials. The fleece could still be used as throws. They would still get a lot of use since my kids like to cuddle up in them even when they are not in bed.

My husband and I also had a queen-size fleece blanket that we used frequently but I didn't know the status of the flame retardant/flammability of that one, so I switched it out for a cotton blanket to go with our cotton duvet until it was cold enough for our down comforter. We had two levels of down blanket, one lighter than the other, both purchased more than 10 years ago. The heavier one never got used because we got extremely overheated every time we tried it out. The lighter one kept us warm enough even when our bedroom got down to 55°F at night. In the end, I ordered a hypoallergenic down comforter for my son with an organic cotton duvet cover since his room was the coldest in the house. I had just finished making a 100% cotton quilt for my daughter for her birthday, so I replaced her fleece with that and added an additional cotton blanket for when it was colder out.

I had a huge amount of trouble trying to find a down throw with a cotton cover for use during the day, so I ended up getting some down throws with polyester covers on them. They aren't toxic or sprayed, so at least I didn't feel like I was violating that rule, but I did feel bad about not getting all-natural materials. Admittedly, it wasn't much of an improvement over the fleece, but I bought them more for one of the challenges that I run on my blog every year rather than for this project. This was the fourth year of my annual "Freeze Yer Buns Challenge" which encouraged people to keep their homes at a cooler temperature during the winter to save energy (*à la* Jimmy Carter and his sweaters) as well as to reduce our carbon footprint.

Since we kept the house temperature at 62°F during the day and 55°F at night, it could get cold if you were just sitting around—which is why we had the extra blankets in the main living space. Additionally, our basement got cold, even during summer, so we had a stack of blankets down there to use as well. The two down throws I bought (mostly because they were on sale) were to be used in the basement, too. At the very least, we no longer used any blanket that had any kind of flame retardant in or on it.

Pining for pajamas

Children's pajamas sold in the United States and intended for kids aged 6 months to 14 years have to be flame resistant. Them's the rules set forth by the Consumer Product Safety Commission (CPSC), like it or not. I didn't like it. It bothered me to no end that I couldn't find kids' pajamas that didn't have flame retardants in them unless you went way out of your way to find them. One exception was pajamas that were tight-fitting. My daughter, who would much rather have something more relaxed and girly *would* wear the form-fitting pajamas. In fact, she's pretty indifferent to a lot of clothing choices as long as they aren't *too* tight. Of course, she certainly had her preferences, but she's somewhat flexible. My son, on the other hand, was not. He has some serious clothing requirements that all stem from his sensory processing and OCD issues. A lot of it was comfort-based and had to do with tags, labels or scratchiness. But a lot of it was also based more on routine and control and what made him comfortable in a security blanket sort of way. We had that problem with all of his clothing, but we didn't push him too hard on it. Even when my mom declared on Christmas morning that he looked like a homeless kid with his well-worn outfit.

When it came time to choose new pajamas for the year, Emma was all excited about the ones I showed her. The 100% organic cotton, form-fitting girlie patterns were fine by her. And the form-fitting design fit the standards as flame resistant. Henry, however, was intent on getting the loose-fitting fleece ones that had the button-down top. Like an adult pair of pajamas. Apparently, it's called "coat style." Unfortunately, since they all were made out of polyester and were always loose-fitting, they were made of flame-resistant fabric. There were plenty of hints online suggesting methods of reducing the flame-retardant chemicals in kids' pajamas by washing them in this or that and following some witches' brew or reciting a few PDBE removal chants, but really they all ended up being just soap with enzymes instead of detergent. Initially I thought the fabric was sprayed with the chemicals, but it turned out the material was treated even before it is woven. So it's quite a bit more difficult to remove than you would think at first. I wasn't interested in trying to remove the flame retardants because I wasn't sure how effective that actually was but I still wanted to keep my kids safe.

If I wasn't going to be able to get Henry form-fitting pajamas because I knew he wouldn't ever wear them, then I was going to have to make another compromise and get him the kind he actually would wear. That is, the pajamas that were flame resistant. It took me weeks to finally come to this conclusion, mostly because I was so hell-bent on trying to remove everything potentially toxic from our environment. But there really wasn't going to be an easy solution with this one. I didn't want to have him wear (non-pajama) loose-fitting clothes that were comfortable for him both physically and mentally but were a potential fire hazard. In either case, there was some risk. I decided I would rather he was exposed to the PBDEs because I couldn't live with myself if we had a fire and he was injured because I chose to dress him in unsafe clothing.

Many parents will buy sweatpants for their children instead of pajamas, since they aren't made of flame-resistant material, and have them sleep in a long shirt. Or they will opt for something like thermal underwear, but not as tight-fitting as the pajamas. It was certainly an option, so before I went out and invested in some flame-resistant pajamas, I asked Henry what he wanted. I knew he loved wearing thermal cotton shirts at one point, so I probably could get him interested in some for bed. They were cotton and form-fitting and were of little risk. The deal-breaker was most likely going to be the pants. He had some older, form-fitting ones whose material I was unsure of since the tags were long gone and there was no way to check, but maybe getting him used to the feel again would make him more amenable to trying the form-fitting pajama sets. I knew he refused to wear sweatpants for whatever reason — I don't know if it was the binding at the bottom or what. For a while, a few years ago, that's all he would wear, though. He gets on these clothing kicks where he *has* to wear a certain item or he feels really uncomfortable in a "freaking out" sort of way. It didn't matter in the end in either case. He wanted nothing to do with them. We ended up getting him the flame-resistant pajamas he desperately wanted.

Avoiding Robespierre

The battle over the flame-resistant fabrics was pissing me off to no end. It had little to do with internal arguments and everything to do with an inability to find alternatives. I couldn't get over how obsequious the whole textile industry was in following the CPSC requirement of flame-retardant material in anything that could remotely be considered children's sleepwear. Robes, for example. I understood that it's a federal requirement and that the standards required that sleepwear, including robes, must be flame resistant, and if the garment ignited, the flame must self-extinguish. But, really, who wears a robe to sleep in? If they were going to be that nutty about it then why not t-shirts and sweats and, frankly, anything you wear because I guarantee you, if you can wear it, you can sleep in it.

Because we were doing the Freeze Yer Buns Challenge for my blog, the house was a tad bit nippy in the morning. The kids saw that my husband was wearing a robe early one morning and they were immensely interested in it. More because it's white and it looked like a karate *gi* and they had karate fantasies in mind. But I did ask them if they wanted me to pick them up some robes to wear in the morning rather than curling up in blankets on those days and times it was still chilly in the house. They were both excited about it and the idea passed the litmus test when they asked about them again the following day without me prompting them.

So I went on a search for kids' robes at the store. I didn't think I would be able to find any store-bought robes made of natural materials, but I thought at the very least that I could find some that weren't covered in toxins. I was wrong. At the time, I didn't know that robes were part of the federal requirement regarding children's sleepwear and flame resistance. Knowing that I wouldn't be able to readily find a robe for my kids at either department stores or chain stores, I went searching online for organic robes.

Fortunately, I found a plethora of them. Unfortunately, they were expensive. I kept looking and found the product segment known as bathrobes, which apparently don't have the same stringent regulations applied to them. It's really all about how an item was marketed. If a robe was sold in the sleepwear section (or could be, I suppose) and might, however unrealistically, be considered as sleepwear, then it must be flame resistant. If, however, it's sold as a bathrobe and not, ostensibly, used as sleepwear, then it's okay, flames and all. After all that searching, I never got around to buying any robes and the kids didn't seem to notice or care.

Blow me

I have relatively wavy hair, but it's really curly around my face. If I try to blow-dry it using a brush it turns into a giant fuzz ball halo around my head. If I want it to lie flat, I have to use a flat iron and straighten it into submission. If I want it to be curly, I have to use curling cream products and a diffuser and let it partially air-dry. I spent years perfecting which products I needed to achieve whichever hairstyle I was rocking for the day. If I try letting it go au naturel or even look at it with a brush in hand, it has more of a Rosanne Rosannadanna thing going on that I'm not too happy about.

About eight months before beginning the project, when I began research for this book, I started eliminating certain hairstyling products from my arsenal of tools because of the questionable ingredients in them. They read like a laundry list of toxins and I decided I should try to limit my exposure to them, even if it was just in my hair. They made contact with my skin when I put it on and I was probably breathing the contaminants in when I dried my hair. Plus, I was probably also breathing the product in just by virtue of the fact that my hair is next to my face and the product probably flaked off during the course of the day. The big issue with the products was really the parabens and the fragrances as well as a number of other ingredients. Unfortunately, at the time, I couldn't find any natural alternative that worked as well. Couple the lack of decent styling products with the fact that I was experimenting off and on with various "natural" shampoos and conditioners and the result was that my hair was a mess.

The most disastrous experiment that I subjected my hair and scalp to, many months previous to this project, was the shampoo, or rather lack of it, called "no poo." Many women and men have successfully used this technique to wash their hair. "No poo" consists of a mixture of baking soda and water with a vinegar rinse, if you were so inclined. You make a paste or liquid of the baking soda and water and rub it into your hair. Theoretically this should work to some degree. Soap is essentially a mixture of fats, acids and base. When you combine baking soda and vinegar and apply them to your greasy scalp, you are mimicking soap to some degree. At least that's what I kept telling myself.

The "no poo" movement is very big in environmental circles for a variety of reasons. Not only is it inexpensive but there is also no plastic packaging and little in the way of the harsh detergents and toxins that generally make up shampoos and conditioners. In the spirit of trying something new, I had decided to give it a whirl and began the regimen knowing full well that there was an adjustment period. This adjustment period is what put me off so long from trying it in the first place because many people reported having extremely greasy, disgusting hair for a month before the "no poo" technique kicked in and their hair felt clean. The claim is that it takes that long for your scalp to adjust to less cleansing and to "decide" that it doesn't need to produce as much oil as when you are washing it with synthetic detergents. This reasoning sounded suspect to me since oil production is determined by hormones and a number of other genetic factors, not some feedback loop with the air and the universe. In spite of all.this, I decided, what the hell, I should shut my mouth and give it a try.

One other thing that made me wary of this experiment was that, by nature, I have very greasy hair. It's genetic, it runs in the family and there's little I can do about it. My hair is greasy hours after I wash it. If I don't wash it every day it gets questionable. Skipping a day is semi-tolerable. Anything longer than that and I would start scaring small children. And husbands. So it was with bated breath that I took the plunge.

It started off a little uncomfortable. I made the mistake of pre-mixing a squeeze bottle filled with the baking soda and water mixture. I figured it would save me time in the shower. I did the same thing with the vinegar. Because a lot of people complained about the vinegar smell in their hair during the day, they suggested steeping some sort of herb in there. I decided to soak some cinnamon sticks and other spices in the vinegar to reduce the salad-dressing hair issue. Unfortunately, what this meant was that I ended up pouring ice-cold solutions onto my hair in order to proceed. Not a good start.

I was somewhat initially impressed at the fact that my scalp felt clean and that, when I dried my hair, it started out kind of sticky wet but then, poof, was miraculously dry all of a sudden. That first day, my hair didn't look dirty, but it didn't look exactly clean either. It had the faint smell of vinegar for most of the day, but I chalked that up to not enough rinsing. The second day, my hair looked clean, but the ends were turning into a tangled mess. I asked my husband to give me the sniff test and he merely declared that I smelled like I just got back from going running. I didn't exactly take that as a positive. As the week wore on, I noticed my scalp got more and more itchy and I had to concentrate to prevent myself from scratching.

By the third day, things still weren't looking up. When I went to wash my hair, it smelled like I was washing hot, fetid bacon. As I was drying it, I noticed my scalp was looking cleanish, but my hair had turned into a giant grease ball. The baking soda was cleaning my scalp, but since I had very long hair, it wasn't making it past the top. The hair from the top of my ears down was filmy and impossible to brush. For the rest of the day, my head itched like crazy and smelled like rotten bacon. Needless to say, I went back to my regular shampoo the following day. It took my hair a while to recover from that experiment.

The other shampoo experiment I tried was using shampoo bars, and I even went so far as to make my own. Shampoo bars are not too dissimilar from regular bath soap, except that they contain jojoba oil and castor oil for conditioning and better lathering, respectively. Water, lye, some base oils and essential oils are pretty much the extent of the ingredients. The large batch that I made lasted about eight months. My husband and kids still use store-bought shampoo bars. My problem with the shampoo bars (homemade or bought from the store) was that, initially, I was being dumb and not conditioning my hair, too. The bars do a fantastic job of cleaning your hair but, given the length of my hair, I needed to find a heavy-duty conditioner.

After the "no poo" experiment, my hair was pretty dried out. That, coupled with the fact that I had stopped using all those helpful, albeit chemical-laden styling products, meant my hair wasn't cooperating anymore. I couldn't get it to curl to save my life and I couldn't get it to stay flat, even after flat-ironing it. It looked stringy and weird, especially in the pieces that frame my face, the ones that have the most curl. So, what's a girl to do with damaged hair? Cut it off. I didn't cut my hair short, I just gave myself some bangs because that was the area that was most uncooperative, curly and damaged. It solved the problem for a while, but I was still wishing it would lie flat. That's when I received the coupon that temporarily changed my life.

The salon where I used to get my hair cut and highlighted was an Aveda salon from which I used to get email updates with discounts and coupons and the like. This particular email coupon included a discount for a new hair treatment called the Brazilian Blowout, a temporary hair-straightening procedure that was touted as being new and improved, all-natural (made from keratin, just like your hair!) and formaldehyde-free. I had heard some really nasty things about straightening treatments in the past, not only because they damaged your hair permanently but also because of the hazardous chemicals used in the treatment itself. So, I really perked up when I saw this coupon and couldn't believe that my Aveda salon, known for its greener products, would offer such a service if it didn't live up to its standards. That's when I went on a major fact-finding mission. Even though I had a deep discount on the service, I wasn't going to spend a couple hundred dollars on poisoning myself. From what I read, the new and improved product was now formaldehyde-free. The previous formula had caused people's eyes to sting and water, and generally smelled terrible. The results, however, were infamous as far as achieving sleek, straight hair without a flat iron.

This updated version of the Brazilian Blowout was supposed to give the same results as the original version *and* was supposed to be good for your hair. According to the product literature, after a few months the treatment wore away, unlike other straightening products that permanently changed the texture of your hair. In other words, it was marketed as a coating that eventually wore off and, in the meantime, made your hair healthier. Better yet, it didn't stink or cause negative health effects and was formaldehyde-free! I believed it all since that's what they were advertising and, again, my Aveda salon was offering the service, so it must be all good. It was a new and improved formula, right?

I was still hesitant at this point but mostly due to the cost. I managed to justify the expense because we were about to leave on a three-week summer trip to the hot and humid east coast and the last thing I wanted was to lug around a hair dryer and a flat iron to deal with my still-frizzled mess of hair. I also managed to justify the expense by calculating how much time I spent fiddling with my hair each day, trying to coax it into something less shocking, versus how much my time was worth. It was all numerical *legerdemain*, but it worked out nonetheless and I made the appointment.

I was nervous when I went in to get the Brazilian Blowout not because I didn't know what to expect, but because I wasn't sure if it would work. The process itself was simple. I asked the stylist why they charge so much for the procedure since it really just consists of painting on the product, blow-drying it, flat-ironing and washing it out. Not surprisingly, the expense had more to do with the product cost because it didn't take that much more time than a hair coloring, which is far less expensive and requires far more skill.

The product didn't smell when it was being applied, but it did burn my scalp. Every time the stylist painted on a new section, my scalp would burn for about 30 seconds and then the sensation would go away. Other than that I didn't notice any problems — no eye stinging or breathing issues. One of the stylists who was helping dry my hair (the stuff is thick and takes forever to dry so I had two people working on my head to save time) was complaining that her eyes were stinging. She hadn't worked with the treatment before and the other stylist suggested she blow-dry my hair away from her face which reduced the problem for her. So, while the fumes weren't really bothering anyone's lungs, it did sting her eyes.

Other than the burning and stinging part it was relatively easy and, I have to admit, the results were amazing. My hair could be blow-dried or air-dried and it would be silky straight. No more frizz and poof for me. Except there was *one* fairly big trade-off. All that scalp burning I experienced during the application didn't just amount to nothing. No. My scalp peeled like crazy for about a month after I had the Brazilian Blowout done. It flaked off in huge chunks. At first, I couldn't figure out what was going on, but then I remembered the scalp irritation and it all made sense. I had never had problems with dandruff before, even during all my "special" shampoo experiments, so I knew it had to be the Blowout. And, in spite of its living up to its super-smooth claims, it was unlikely I would ever spend that amount of money on it again.

Therefore, I wasn't too surprised when, in late October, as I was ending the second month of my book project, I read a post on

NPR's website reporting how a stylist in Oregon was experiencing health problems after starting to offer the Brazilian Blowout service.[39] Concerned about what was happening to her, she contacted the Oregon Health & Science University's Center for Research on Occupational & Environmental Toxicology. They tested samples of the product (labeled "formaldehyde-free") not only from her salon but also from other salons in Oregon providing the service. Their results showed that the formaldehyde levels in the product were between 8.85% and 10.6%, which is far higher than the 0.2% that is considered safe by the Cosmetic Ingredient Review Panel.

Later testing by Health Canada, a Canadian federal government agency, revealed 12% formaldehyde in the solution, prompting the agency to work toward stopping distribution of the product in Canada.[40] Health Canada stated that the negative physical reactions were being caused by the formaldehyde becoming aerosolized during the blow-drying and flat-ironing part of the service. The manufacturer of Brazilian Blowout still maintains that the product is safe, and that it contains low levels or, at the very least, safe levels of formaldehyde. This is, at least, a turnaround from previous claims that the product was formaldehyde-free.

There was a serious amount of backpedaling and denial going on by the manufacturer, as there should be given the false advertising. They either erroneously or purposefully were marketing their product to be something that it was not. It's bad enough that there are multitudes of products out there with dangerous, carcinogenic ingredients in them and we certainly don't need additional ones flat-out lying about the ingredient content. Also, not too surprising is the fact that a class action lawsuit was filed against the manufacturer not too long after the results of the testing by Oregon and Health Canada hit the news. As of this writing, salons in my area were still offering the service.

Licking the windowsills

The test results from my labs started to trickle in at the tail end of October. The first one was an email from Anatek Labs explaining the results of the bacterial test I had ordered of our home drinking water. While not necessarily a toxin or a contaminant in the same category of everything else I was testing, I figured that, since I was having the drinking water tested, I'd throw the bacteria test in for fun as well. I was happy to read that the test for coliform bacteria came back negative. Because it was negative, there was no need for any further tests to see what kinds of colonies of bacteria were lurking in my water. I was so excited by the news that I posted it on my Facebook wall. This goes to show that I probably need to get out of the house more often.

The next test result I received was a rather cryptic email from Anatek Labs regarding the lead paint sample I sent in with a note saying "This is not considered lead paint." After a few emails back and forth and after viewing the lab result itself, I managed to suss out a few more details. The hunk of paint I scraped from the wall behind Emma's bedroom door tested in at 176 mg/Kg of lead.

Since I'm a pessimist and certified hypochondriac, that sounded like a heck of a lot of lead to me. However, after looking at some information from the EPA and confirming it with the lab, I deduced that, if the lab report is expressed as a weight (which it was), then the federal definition of lead-based paint is 0.5% lead, which is the same as 5,000 mg/Kg of lead.[41] And 176 mg/Kg is not quite as high as 5,000 mg/Kg. So maybe our paint didn't have as much lead as I initially thought and, basically, anything less than 5,000 mg/Kg of lead is not considered to be lead paint. Since our sample wasn't even close to the threshold or even in the ballpark, I was pretty relieved to see that all those years of not dusting the paint particles off the windowsills in the kids' bedrooms wasn't contributing to any lead poisoning.

Pure as the driven snow

About a week after I got the lead paint lab report, I received the results of our water testing in the mail. Since the city water coming into the house was, relatively speaking, rather excellent in terms of contaminants, I wasn't too worried about the water results in spite of my penchant for catastrophic thinking. I did have some fears about lead and some other heavy metals and I wasn't too happy with the fluoride levels in our water supply as well as the chlorine smell in the water, but a good water filter could help out with that.

In any case, some of the nastier things like arsenic, cadmium and mercury came back ND, or not detected. Nothing was anywhere near the EPA's maximum contaminant levels (MCL). The lead came in at 0.00210 mg/L where the MCL is 0.015 mg/L. In fact, all the results were minuscule in comparison to the EPA's maximum levels. I was somewhat surprised to also see that our fluoride level was 0.881 mg/L since the testing at the treatment plant puts it at 1.04 mg/L. The EPA limits set fluoride at 4.0 mg/L due to the inherent health issues mentioned above.

All in all, our water results came back with a fantastic thumbs-up, but I still used the drinking water filter since I wanted to remove the chlorine and its smell and taste as well as even more of the fluoride. If our filter truly did remove 65% of the fluoride as advertised then that would put our fluoride levels in the water at about 0.3 mg/L. As for the copper, that came back really low, so I don't know what was causing the blue-green staining on the porcelain in our tub. It was certainly not from high levels of any metal but may be a result of long-term exposure to other minerals in the water. Even though I didn't specifically test for them, a lot of the other contaminants that were tested by the city came back as not detected by their labs so it wasn't as important to filter them out, even though our filter would have if they were present. When I got the lab results back, I became a little less anal retentive about using only filtered water because our home drinking water appeared to be about as pure as the driven snow. And for that, I'm grateful.

Parabens and phthalates results

Emma and I were still lacking a Halloween costume about five days before the main event. She had a Halloween party scheduled in her classroom a few days before Halloween and we were cutting it close on the costume. Henry had decided to reuse his costume from the year before in exchange for the money that it would cost to buy him a new one so he could get a new Lego set. Of course, the amount we gave him was at a substantial discount on the cost of an actual new costume, but he was happy even with the creative financing going on.

In any case, as Emma and I were pulling in to the parking lot at our neighborhood Value Village for costume ideas, I got a call on my cell phone from Dr. Hibbs to let me know that he had received my lab test results for the phthalate and paraben profiles and that one of the phthalates and two of the parabens were very high.

On one hand I was giddy that I was finally getting something to work with. Not that I wanted to be contaminated or anything, but after the lead paint and water test results came back sparkling, it was nice to know that these contaminants — ones that were a little easier to manipulate — were the ones coming in high. On the other hand, it really surprised me how high they were given the products I was using at the time I did the lab tests. I had been using some natural products mixed in with more mainstream stuff. If my body was so chock-full of parabens and phthalates, what did it mean for the average person who uses all conventional products with complete disregard to ingredient labels?

What does it mean?

Before I go over the initial set of test results for parabens and phthalates, there are some things I need to point out about the different populations that I'm comparing my test results to. The Environmental Working Group (EWG)/Commonweal studies noted below were done using the same sampling method I used — using first morning urine. The CDC biomonitoring group had their urine sample collected at random times of the day, which is why their results are lower since there is less concentration in the urine. To more accurately compare the results, then, I think it's fair to focus on the EWG results to see how I measured up. Even with looking at the EWG/Commonweal results, you can see that my numbers far exceed the geometric mean in their studies. I think it's also fair to say that my numbers are particularly high.

First up…the phthalates group. Now, this is some seriously sloggy reading, but it will go quickly, so bear with me for a page or two. All of the following information was derived from the Environmental Working Group's Human Toxome Project: Mapping the Pollution in People.

MEtP

The one phthalate for which I tested very high (and was flagged on the report) was *monoethyl phthalate* MEtP, a breakdown product of diethyl phthalate (DEP),which is used in perfume, cologne, deodorant, soap, shampoo, lotion and other personal care products, particularly those containing fragrance. Animal studies have shown that DEP causes toxicity of the liver and kidneys as well as altered pituitary, adrenal, thyroid, brain and heart weight. Developmental exposure can cause skeletal abnormalities. A 2007 study showed that, aside from causing reproductive impairments in utero, increased levels of MEtP, the metabolite of DEP, was associated with increased waist circumference and insulin resistance in adult men in the United States.[42]

So, how did my test results of MEtP compare to other studies done on the general population in the U.S.?[43] Not very good at all.

EWG/Commonweal results
58 μg/g creatinine in urine (geometric mean)
found in 74 out of 74 of the people tested

CDC biomonitoring results
166 μg/g creatinine in urine (geometric mean)
found in 7,922 of the 8,015 people tested

Deanna Duke's results
>2,500 μg/g creatinine in urine
95% reference interval ≤3,143 μg/g creatinine in urine

---

mEHHP and mEHP

The second-highest phthalate test result was for mono-(2-ethyl-5-hydroxyhexyl) phthalate (mEHHP). Both mEHHP and mono-(2-ethylhexyl)phthalate (mEHP) are metabolites, or breakdown products, of bis(2-ethylhexyl)phthalate, aka DEHP. DEHP is used in soft plastic, especially PVC, and is also sometimes present in clear food wrap, personal care products, medical devices, detergents and soaps, and pesticides. I hoped that the results of this test were due to personal care products and soaps and not from anything else since consumer products are easier to eliminate and I could, therefore, reduce my exposure.

According to the Environmental Working Group, "exposure to DEHP occurs through direct use of products containing this chemical, consumption of foods wrapped in products containing this chemical, and through inhalation of air contaminated with this chemical." Studies done by the CDC show that measurements of mEHHP in the urine of more than 2,500 Americans indicate that younger children (ages 6–11) are more exposed than older children (ages 12–19) and adults. The European Union has banned DEHP as a result of concerns about exposure as well as toxicity. Studies have shown that in laboratory animals, fetal exposure to DEHP causes significant developmental toxicity, especially of the male reproductive system. In adult animals, DEHP causes cancer and toxicity to the reproductive organs, adrenal gland, liver and kidneys.[44]

How did my tests results for mEHHP and mEHP compare to other studies done on the general population in the U.S.?[45] Still terribly bad.

Table 1.

mEHHP	mEHP
EWG/Commonweal results	
64.8 µg/g creatinine in urine (geometric mean)	8.45 µg/g creatinine in urine (geometric mean)
found in 74 out of 74 of the people tested	found in 64 out of 74 of the people tested
CDC biomonitoring results	
18.4 µg/g creatinine in urine (geometric mean)	2.96 µg/g creatinine in urine (geometric mean)
found in 5,379 of the 5,479 people tested	found in 7,143 of the 8,020 people tested

mEHHP	mEHP
Deanna Duke's results	
255 µg/g creatinine in urine	36 µg/g creatinine in urine
95% reference interval ≤1,253 µg/g creatinine in urine	95% reference interval ≤209 µg/g creatinine in urine

mEOHP

Rounding out the phthalates list was mono-(2-ethyl-5-oxohexyl) phthalate (mEOHP). This is also a metabolite of DEHP with exposure and toxicity occurring in the same way as with mEHP and mEHHP. The latest exposure study from the Centers for Disease Control indicates that mEOHP is a widespread contaminant of the human body. Measurements of mEOHP in the urine of more than 2,500 Americans indicate that women are slightly more exposed than men, and younger children (ages 6–11) are more exposed than older children (ages 12–19) and adults.

How did my tests results for mEOHP compare to other studies done on the general population in the U.S.?[46] Could have been worse, but not too miserable.

EWG/Commonweal results
39.4 µg/g creatinine in urine (geometric mean)
found in 73 out of 74 of the people tested

CDC biomonitoring results
12.7 µg/g creatinine in urine (geometric mean)
found in 5,364 of the 5,479 people tested

Deanna Duke's results
74 µg/g creatinine in urine
95% reference interval ≤569 µg/g creatinine in urine

Now, on to the parabens.

Propylparaben

This particular paraben tested scary high. Even higher than the 95% reference interval given by Metametrix. In general, parabens are thought to mimic estrogen and, in turn, may contribute to estrogen-stimulated breast cancers. Research from a 2002 study found that doses of propylparaben increased the growth and gene expression of estrogen-sensitive breast cancer cells, responses similar to those provoked by a potent form of estrogen known as estradiol. In 2004, a study testing for parabens in breast cancer tumors found propylparaben in 15 of 20 tumors.

It's not just breast tissue that's up for grabs with parabens either. Animal studies indicate that propylparaben has other hormone-disrupting effects as well. Studies exposing young rats to propylparaben in food led to reduced sperm and testosterone production in males, even at "acceptable" levels.[47]

How did my tests results of propylparaben compare to other studies done on the general population in the U.S.?[48] As I said above, scary.

EWG/Commonweal results
11.2 µg/g creatinine in urine (geometric mean)
found in 26 out of 28 of the people tested

Deanna Duke's results
>2,500 µg/g creatinine in urine
95% reference interval ≤959 µg/g creatinine in urine

Methylparaben and ethylparaben

Not unlike propylparaben, methylparaben and ethylparaben have some problems of their own. Studies show that both have weak hormone-disrupting characteristics, causing concern that they may contribute to estrogen-stimulated breast cancers. A 2004 study testing for parabens in human breast cancer tumors found methylparaben in 19 of 20 tumors and ethylparaben in 16 of 20 tumors. Recent research has found that doses of methylparaben and ethylparaben trigger growth responses in estrogen-sensitive breast cancer cells as well.[49]

How did my tests results of methylparaben[50] and ethylparaben[51] compare to other studies done on the general population in the U.S.? Still crappy, indeed.

EWG/Commonweal results — methylparaben

77.7 µg/g creatinine in urine (geometric mean)

found in 28 out of 28 of the people tested

Deanna Duke's results — methylparaben

>2,500 µg/g creatinine in urine

95% reference interval ≤2,995 µg/g creatinine in urine

EWG/Commonweal results — ethylparaben

1.61 µg/g creatinine in urine (geometric mean)

found in 21 out of 28 of the people tested

Deanna Duke's results — ethylparaben

78 µg/g creatinine in urine

95% reference interval ≤282 µg/g creatinine in urine

Butylparaben

Similar to methyl and ethylparabens, butylparaben has estrogenic effects. And, as with propylparaben, animal studies indicate that butylparaben has other hormone-disrupting effects as well. Exposing young rats and mice to butylparaben in food led to reduced sperm and testosterone production and other negative reproductive health effects in males, even at "acceptable" levels. Injections of isobutylparaben were also shown to increase mouse uterus weight, a further indication of hormone activity. The estrogenicity of butylparaben appears to be greater because of its larger chemical size in comparison to smaller chemicals like methylparaben; in addition, the branched, or iso-, form of butylparaben may be more estrogenic.

How did my tests results of butylparaben compare to other studies done on the general population in the U.S.?[52] Slightly better than the other paraben tests.

EWG/Commonweal results

0.744 µg/g creatinine in urine (geometric mean)

found in 18 out of 28 of the people tested

Deanna Duke's results

3 µg/g creatinine in urine

95% reference interval ≤ 36 µg/g creatinine in urine

What on Earth was I using?

The body products I was using before I took the parabens and phthalates urine test consisted of a "sensitive skin" sunblock with a variety of parabens, a body lotion with parabens, hair shampoo and conditioner with parabens, and makeup with possibly some parabens. All of these products (except for the sunblock) contained the ingredient "fragrance," which most likely meant there were some phthalates in them as well, but they do not get listed as such. The body soap I used had fragrance in it and the Chanel nail polish had some phthalates derivative in there as well.

Since the sunblock was supposed to be for sensitive skin it was allegedly fragrance-free and hypoallergenic. It did, however, contain some suspicious sunscreen chemicals and a few different parabens as well.[53] The body lotion I used was from the Alba brand and was considered to be a "natural" product. With a name like Alba Organics Hawaiian Kona Coffee Lotion, you wouldn't think it would have parabens in it. But it did (methylparabens and polyparabens to be exact). The shampoo and conditioner that I used, both from Biolage, give the impression that they are natural and made from botanical ingredients, which they are, but they also contain a number of sketchy ingredients. Both products work fantastically—but at a cost. The company branding for Biolage advertises a concern for the environment but, apparently, not as much for their customer's health.

The upside to these terrible lab results was that I hoped that the elimination of these products would drastically reduce my numbers. After discussing these contaminants with Dr. Hibbs, my initial understanding of how the body processes parabens and phthalates wasn't exactly as I initially thought. It's true that they are all generally processed by the body and eliminated within 24–48 hours, but, and I guess this should not have surprised me, some of the chemicals still get stored in the body, mostly in body fat. It would be entirely possible to get misleading results in my follow-up tests if those stored parabens and phthalates are still being released from my fat into my waste stream. In this case, the follow-up urine test might show detectable levels of these chemicals in my system even though I'm no longer being exposed to them.

At that point, I immediately ceased using all those products. Any temptation to cheat and use them or any other conventional product was squashed when I thought of those lab results. When I saw a commercial or an ad for the latest personal care or beauty product or wished I could use one of my favorite "old" products, I just reminded myself of how high the parabens and phthalates were in my body and there was no way I could justify adding more. I would just have to find replacement products that I loved just as much (or worked nearly as well) that didn't contain potentially dangerous chemicals.

Halloween: What actually happened

Back at Value Village, after I talked to Dr. Hibbs about my lab results, Emma found a Halloween costume she liked. She ended up picking out a pre-packaged costume with a spider queen theme. It is funny how, even at age seven, kids worry about what other kids think. After we bought the costume, she was concerned that the other kids in her class wouldn't like it. I think she was relieved when she saw a third grader wearing the same costume at their school Halloween party. I ended up renting a costume when my husband decided he wanted to go to a costume rental shop. Mine definitely didn't have any chemicals in it, just cotton, as did my husband's.

For some reason, Halloween 2010 seemed to be the year when news stories about the flammability of Halloween costumes hit the media big time. Maybe this happens every year and I just never paid attention to it before but I, frankly, wasn't aware of this issue until my mom warned us to keep the kids away from lit Halloween pumpkins because of the flammability issue. She watches the news like crazy so she was our sentinel into Flammability Fears 2010. According to the news, the Consumer Product Safety Commission was telling parents to look for flame-resistant costumes without baggy sleeves, long capes or billowing skirts that could catch fire on a nearby candle. In fact, some media outlets were sharing recipes on how to makes clothes flame resistant naturally, by using a mixture of borax and water. I would take this combo any day over chemical flame-resistant materials.

Most apparel has information listed about the materials used and, since I knew the brand of Henry's costume, I looked it up online. It was made out of polyester and hard plastic and didn't appear to be classified as flame resistant. In retrospect, I think Emma's costume was made of flame-resistant materials but I didn't see anything on the packaging. After a little bit of digging, I found out that all costumes sold in the U.S. used to be flame resistant as per the Flammable Fabrics Act of 1953, but textile manufacturers are no longer required by law to make costumes flame retardant.[54]

Emma's costume may have been made out of 100% polyester and not contain flame retardant, but I no longer had the packaging and couldn't find it online, so I'll never know. If it did, however, this sucked and not just for the holiday itself. When you add in the fact that kids tend to wear their costumes year round, regardless of the occasion, it just means that they are exposed to these chemicals far more often than you think. Sleeping. Playing dress-up. Cozying up in a robe. How much of their day is spent in flame-resistant clothing or PVC? One little surprise that I didn't anticipate was that the goggles that came with Henry's costume were made out of PVC.[55] He fortunately broke the foam mask that came with the costume the previous year, but he did like to wear the goggles for a variety of reasons. Even though he didn't wear them for trick-or-treating on his eyes that night (it was too dark) he still wore them on his head. And he wore them on his face year round for pretend play. I should have suspected the goggles were made out of PVC given the plastic, but I didn't look up the material contents until after the fact.

At least our exposure to Halloween decorations ended up being minimal. For some reason, my kids had no interest in decorating the house or the front yard that year. In years past, they would have me out there decorating the house weeks before Halloween and, in one year, in mid-August. I tell you I was never so happy to put away the decorations after looking at them for over two months. I don't know what the problem was this time around, but the end result was that the only decorations we put up were two metal and wood signs and some carved pumpkins with soy candles. No toxins there.

The candy we handed out was all either packaged in foil or in little waxed boxes. It's certainly possible there was some nonstick coating in there somewhere but, short of not handing out candy, it was the best we could find given the information I had. However, the candy my kids hauled home had some nonstick wrappers. Emma didn't have too much as she only made it to about five houses before the neighbor's motion-sensor smoke machine scared the crap out of her and she headed back to the homestead. Henry acquired a bit more loot, but I wasn't going to be the parent who took away their Halloween candy. I suppose we could have done a candy trade—I'll give you one organic, non-toxic donut for two Teflon Tasties—but I didn't want to traumatize them any more than necessary. It wasn't worth the fight and, oh boy, it would have been a fight.

To wrap up Halloween—it was a semi-fail on the costumes and incoming candy, but a big non-toxic win on the decorations, candles and outgoing candy.

Heavy metal lab results

When I received the photocopies of the parabens and phthalates results in the mail about a week later, Dr. Hibbs had also snuck in copies of the heavy metal lab results from the two tests I had taken a few weeks back. The first set of results was from the blood test that included nutrient elements like calcium, magnesium, zinc and copper, as well as potentially toxic elements such as arsenic, cadmium, lead, mercury, uranium and a host of other goodies. The second test was from the 24-hour urine collection which focused mostly on toxic elements like aluminum, antimony, cesium, tungsten and the same ones mentioned above. The results for both sets of tests left me somewhat confused but, on the whole, there wasn't anything too frightening in them.

Whole blood results for metals

The copies of the lab results included not only the resulting numbers, but also the reference range, percentiles and a summary, explaining what was too high or too low. For the nutrient elements, my magnesium, calcium, copper, zinc, manganese, selenium and strontium values were all within the normal range. There were only two standouts in this test. The first one that was flagged was the nutrient element lithium—my levels were lower than they should have been.

Lithium salts are well known as being used as a treatment for bipolar disorder as well as a number of other mental diseases. Lithium is a soft, silver-white metal commonly found in oceans and all living organisms. This nutrient element apparently serves a biological function but plants and animals can survive fine without it. However, maybe if I had higher lithium levels I'd be happier and bouncier. You can buy over-the-counter nonprescription lithium supplements, but I never got around to finding out if taking lithium supplements would be a good idea for me.

The second nutrient element flagged was something called molybdenum, which I had never heard of before and still can't pronounce without thinking a little too hard about it. Molybdenum can help prevent anemia and is oftentimes used as a supplement since it is thought to have antioxidant properties. Apparently it assists the body by fighting nitrosamines (the breakdown product of nitrates) which can cause cancer. Molybdenum is necessary for normal cell function and the metabolism of nitrogen, and assists in the breakdown of sulfite toxin buildup in the body. People who have a reaction to sulfites in preserved foods (like wine or dried fruit) oftentimes lack sufficient levels of molybdenum, which is a part of sulfite oxidase, the enzyme that helps break down sulfites.[56]

Regardless of its function and unpronouncability, my levels of molybdenum were too high. And by that I mean outside the reference range high. The issue with this nutrient being too high is that it can inhibit the absorption of iron and copper and interfere with the binding of copper to some proteins. However, molybdenum toxicity is rare and, since my copper and iron levels were normal, I decided to ignore this result as well.

In regards to the toxic elements in the whole blood sample, all of the elements tested for fell below the reference range upper limit listed on the lab report. Which is a good thing. To reiterate, the only unusual thing that I did before I had the blood test was get a flu shot a week prior to the blood draw as well as eat a little seafood (and I'm talking small amounts) two days before the draw. Only a few heavy metals showed up as possible standouts, but none of them were flagged in the report.

Arsenic

Arsenic was the toxic element that Dr. Hibbs had warned could show false highs if I ate seafood, so it was entirely possible that the somewhat elevated result was due to that consumption. My follow-up lab test at the end of the project would shed some light on whether or not the elevated level of arsenic was diet induced.

Arsenic is a known human carcinogen, associated with an increased risk of skin, lung, bladder, kidney, liver and colon cancer. Long-term exposures to arsenic can be deadly. Arsenic is also associated with kidney failure, respiratory toxicity, circulation disorders (Raynaud's, blood vessel constriction, cold hands and feet, numbness in hands and feet), cardiological effects (low blood pressure, heart attack, stroke, high heart rate and arrhythmia) and neurotoxicity. Neurological effects of arsenic exposure include peripheral nerve damage, hallucinations, memory loss and agitation.[57]

I didn't have any EWG or CDC numbers to compare this element to, just my own. I had 4.4 μg/L of whole blood with the reference range topping out at 9.0.

Lead

Lead is a big one on everyone's list of "scary" contaminants because it is a highly toxic heavy metal that can cause permanent neurological and behavioral problems (like ADHD) and affects virtually every system in the body. It can also cause developmental defects in children, preterm delivery, low birth weight and fetal growth retardation. Since Henry has neurodevelopmental issues, and was born both preterm and at a low birth weight, I was concerned about my own lead levels and whether or not my exposure could have influenced his development in utero. Given the fact that the amount of lead paint in our current home was low, I had less to fear in general. Our old home, however, the one we lived in when I was pregnant with my kids, was most likely a lead paint bomb. And, since the most common source of lead exposure these days is house paint, it was definitely something to worry about.

Our previous home was a 1916 Craftsman-style home with beautiful wood detailing inside, all of it painted and all of it showing multiple layers of paint buildup from over the years. I doubt that anyone in the past had taken the time to do any lead paint abatement and gotten it removed because it really was almost a geologic record of paint layers, complete with bug bodies trapped in between. With the kids crawling around and sucking on things at the old house, I'm sure some lead was ingested. Hopefully, the amount they got from me when they were fetuses was minimal.

According to the Environmental Working Group, lead can "affect children at extremely low levels, and there is no evidence of a threshold dose below which developmental effects does not occur. Levels as low as 10 micrograms per deciliter, currently considered the threshold for elevated blood lead level, have been associated with decreased intelligence and impaired neurobehavioral development."[58]

So, it was with glee that I compared my lead blood results with those of other individuals. Finally, one of my lab results actually fell lower than the other test subjects.

EWG/Commonweal results
1.37 µg/dL wet weight in whole blood (geometric mean)
found in 73 out of 73 of the people tested

CDC biomonitoring results
1.33 µg/dL wet weight in whole blood (geometric mean)
found in 7,896 of the 8,373 people tested

Deanna Duke's results
0.7 µg/dL wet weight in whole blood (geometric mean)
reference range < 3.0

Mercury

Mercury is another big no-no and we are all told to avoid it like the plague in food, and particularly fish. I eat relatively little tuna but, living in the Pacific Northwest where we enjoy easy access to fresh wild salmon, let's just say that we eat a lot of salmon during the summer and fall. Salmon isn't particularly known for being high in mercury compared to other fish, but it is still a large, fatty fish high on the food chain and bioaccumulation toxins along with the best of them.

My lab test measured a couple of different types of mercury. Metallic mercury (like the stuff found in thermometers, dental fillings and fluorescent lights) was the first type; ethyl mercury (like the thimerosal preservative in my vaccine the week before) was the second; and methyl mercury (the kind found in seafood) was the last. My test results were a resultant mixture of all of those three exposures that I've had over the years. Since mercury, like the rest of the heavy metals, bioaccumulates in your body, the lab results can only show a snapshot of what is circulating in your blood at the time. Your body removes half of any mercury exposure within about two months and the rest of it is stored. If any of the forms of mercury reach the brain, they can be stored there, potentially indefinitely.

I hadn't used a mercury-based thermometer in years and I have never had dental fillings of the metal sort, so my exposure to metallic mercury was, at least recently, low. The more definitive test on any of these heavy metals would have been a fat biopsy to see what's really lurking in there. Most exposure to mercury these days is through seafood consumption, since your stomach absorbs about 95% of the mercury stored in the fish's tissues.[59] Physicians caution pregnant women to slow down or limit their consumption of fish that is considered to be high in mercury because methylmercury is toxic to the developing fetal brain—it can cause a delay of mental development in utero and learning deficiencies. Roughly 10% of U.S. women have mercury levels in their blood that are potentially unsafe for a fetus.[60]

Long-term, low-level exposure to mercury can cause kidney and nerve damage, muscle tremors, irritability, personality changes and gingivitis and is associated with leukemia and possibly liver cancer and chromosomal damage. Methylmercury exposure is also associated with changes in the immune system and kidneys, decreased fertility and possible cardiovascular effects.[61]

How did my mercury levels compare to the rest of humanity? Not terrible, but not great, either. I was still higher than the average.

EWG/Commonweal results
0.737 µg/L wet weight in whole blood (geometric mean)
found in 42 out of 42 of the people tested

CDC biomonitoring results
0.56 µg/L wet weight in whole blood (geometric mean)
found in 7,584 of the 8,373 people tested

Deanna Duke's results
1.0 µg/L wet weight in whole blood
reference range < 5.0 µg/L

Urine test for metals

Just to spice things up, I decided to eat a can of tuna the day before the urine test. It was local, line-caught albacore tuna, so the methylmercury levels would be higher than in nonalbacore tuna.

However, recent studies have shown that albacore caught off the coasts of Washington, Oregon and California have far lower mercury levels than albacore caught elsewhere, so it might not have registered much of anything.[62] Eating tuna could also potentially increase cadmium levels in my urine. Research studies have found that tuna and salmon, both large pelagic fish, have some mercury, lead and cadmium in them. Because levels of these toxins have been found in lower concentrations in our local and Alaskan fish populations, I didn't think it would make much of an impact but I still wanted to try it out and see. The test results showed my mercury levels to be nothing out of the ordinary.

In the rest of the results of my heavy metals urine test there were really only two standouts or, rather, two toxic elements that registered in the elevated zone: tungsten and cadmium. Fire-retardant fabric coatings tend to test high in tungsten although I didn't think I had any clothing that met that description. In any case, most of the tungsten that enters your blood is quickly flushed from your body through your urine. I didn't know the source of my tungsten exposure, but the follow-up lab test may shed some light on that.

The cadmium must not have been much of an issue because it was not flagged in the lab report and my doctor made a note that the number looked fine. Cadmium is a known carcinogen and can cause all manner of tumors and cancers like leukemia, lymphomas and sarcoma. It can also cause emphysema; liver, kidney or pancreas toxicity; skeletal problems and a whole host of other issues. There is not one bodily system it leaves untouched. So, I was glad to see that my cadmium levels weren't remarkable.

Adjusting to Non-toxic Living

Getting my drink on

When I first started this project, I was planning on forgoing all alcoholic beverages for the duration, mostly because I wanted my liver to focus on processing out the toxins in my body rather than working on processing the alcohol. The justification seemed sound to me. Since I was eliminating as much exposure to toxins as possible it would give my body a chance to try to get rid of what was already stored in there. This, coupled with an actual planned detox at the end of the project, as suggested by Dr. Hibbs, would help jolt the remaining toxins out of my body. Or that was the theory. I still wasn't sure how much hidden exposure I was getting from food, air, water and random events like washing my hands in a public restroom.

I mentioned my planned alcohol abstinence to two of my friends, one of whom owns two bars which the other visits frequently. They responded as if I were truly off my rocker. They figured this would be the hardest part of the project. Without going into too much detail, I would heartily disagree. While I like the occasional drink, I can easily forgo it as well. At least, that's what I thought. I knew that I had become a more consistent drinker over the years and I certainly can't argue that a drink in the evening with dinner is something I really enjoy. But I can also skip it without too much of a sacrifice.

In true self-delusional justification, however, I decided it might be worthwhile to actually explore non-toxic drinking. In other words, is it possible to find wine and liquor with few to no toxins in the form of residual pesticides, herbicides and fungicides? Alcohol can be considered inherently toxic in that it taxes your body, but it also provides health benefits, as shown by many recent studies.[1] One of the reasons I don't mind a drink now and again is because I do have migraines and alcohol acts as a blood thinner. Between these benefits and the possible prevention of stroke, I have convinced myself over the years that drinking does more good than harm. More importantly, I wanted to make this project realistic. It's not realistic to expect that there are no other options between drinking conventionally produced alcohol and dropping it all cold turkey. There are too many people who enjoy drinking alcohol, whether it's wine or spirits. I felt it would be more valuable to cover this topic as part of exploring food and drink than to just ignore it altogether. Plus, it would be one of the more enjoyable parts of the project.

One thing I wanted to explore as part of the project was to see how hard it was to find organic wine and liquor. Even though I'd be ignoring the possible liver damage from drinking, I wanted to make sure I wasn't potentially imbibing pesticides and who knows what else from non-organic drinks. With this mission in mind, I went on a search for organic wine as well as replacements for my favorite cocktail ingredients. It ended up being a lot more difficult than I anticipated.

In the last few years, more organic options have come on the market. The problem really is with accessibility and availability. The United States still has a lot of antiquated liquor laws, something akin to Prohibition-lite, I'm afraid, depending on the state where you live. Washington State has the most inane liquor laws, as do many other states in the union. Having lived in California, where you can buy hard alcohol and spirits in the grocery store and the overall costs are considerably lower, dealing with the Washington State Liquor Board's rules has been an annoyance. This annoyance extends not only to establishments that serve liquor, but to pretty much every individual attempting to buy it as well.

If you want to buy something beyond beer and wine you have to go to a Washington state liquor store. These stores only carry limited supplies of liquor and are open limited hours. So, if you are looking for something specific you either have to plan ahead, order a case of it or give up in defeat. In fact, that fall, just as I was trying to locate these elusive organic beverages, there were two separate initiatives on the November ballot trying to dismantle the liquor board and allow other stores to sell liquor. If only we had something like a Beverages & More to loosen the grip on the state-controlled stores, access to organic spirits would be a whole lot easier.

I searched the state liquor board's website to see what organic liquor they did sell and at which stores. I managed to find an organic gin and vodka. There are quite a few organic tequilas manufactured and sold in other areas of the country, but none at my local liquor stores. Even if there were, I generally drink tequila with something like Cointreau or Grand Marnier, so I would have to make my own organic version since there are no organic versions of this orange liqueur sold in this state.

Even though I generally don't drink vodka-based cocktails, I started getting desperate and ended up buying a local organic vodka from Bainbridge Organic Distillers, which is just across the water from us on Puget Sound. They get the grains for their liquors from small organic family farms in Washington State. Since my husband likes gin martinis (when he's not on chemo) and I like gin gimlets, I picked up some organic gin from England. It's a London Dry-style gin called Juniper Green and it was every bit as good as the small craft gin distilleries we have been spoiled by here in the Pacific Northwest. I wanted to try out the Bainbridge Organic gin when the Juniper Green got low, but it's not carried in any of the state's stores.

The one organic tequila sold in the state (Tierras Blanco Organic Tequila) is only available at the Shoreline store, which is about a 20-minute drive north of us. I couldn't exactly justify the drive unless I needed to be up there. But, in the meantime, I decided to make my own triple sec (aka orange liqueur) so that, if I ever got my hands on some organic tequila, I would be able to make an organic margarita. Because it was difficult to find organic spirits and it took planning to make some of my own liqueurs, I

Organic Triple Sec

This recipe is based on the one by Charlie Hodges from the Ace Hotel in Palm Springs that was printed in *Imbibe Magazine*'s Fall 2009 issue. I've specified choosing organic products to make sure that you have a truly non-toxic-produced triple sec.

Ingredients
- 2 small organic navel oranges (preferably Seville oranges)
- 12 oz. organic vodka
- 6 oz. can organic mandarin orange slices*
- 2.5 cups organic cane sugar
- 1.5 cups filtered water

Directions
1. Heat the oven to its lowest temperature setting, generally around 180°F–200°F. Slice the oranges into ⅛-inch-thick wheels and lay them out on a baking tray (preferably not a nonstick tray). Bake the oranges until sticky and gummy but not dried, 1–2 hours.
2. Drain the can of organic mandarin oranges and place them in a jar with 6 oz. of the vodka to infuse for about 24 hours or until it tastes strongly of the oranges.
3. Combine the baked orange slices with the other 6 oz. vodka and infuse for 8 hours, stirring occasionally.
4. Make a simple syrup by combining the sugar and filtered water and stirring over medium heat until dissolved.
5. Finally, strain all the liquid ingredients through a fine sieve and combine with the syrup. Stir and bottle the triple sec. It keeps refrigerated for about a month.

*If you can find Native Forest organic mandarin oranges, use those, as they are the only ones I know of that do not use BPA in the lining of their cans.

drank a lot less and treasured what I had more. Drinking cocktails became more of a special occasion thing because of the difficulty in finding organic versions of the products.

Organic wine

Finding organic wines was a little bit of a challenge as well. Most stores don't carry any organic options and many that do carry them only offer organic wines with no sulfites added. I've tried several no-sulfite wines in the past and I just flat-out don't like them. I find them to be terribly undrinkable. I found one white wine in my grocery store that was made from organically grown grapes, but since it contained added sulfites it could not be labeled as organic. It was very good, but I wanted more than just one option. And preferably something red. I also wanted to find out what the deal was with sulfites and whether or not they were considered toxic at all.

Organic Margarita

This is my favorite recipe for a margarita. I much prefer blanco tequila to an aged one, but it's up to you. There are organic tequilas in blanco, añejo and reposado. I prefer to drink margaritas in a martini glass, but you can use any kind of glass for this.

Ingredients (makes 1)
- ½ small organic lime (cut into quarters)
- Rock salt (for the glass rim, if desired)
- 2 tsp. organic simple syrup (see above)
- 1.5 oz. organic tequila (preferably a blanco)
- 1.5 oz. organic triple sec (see above)

Directions
Muddle the lime in the bottom of a cocktail shaker, removing the lime pieces and squeezing any remaining juice back into the shaker. If you like salt on the rim of your glass, rub one of the lime pieces around the rim and dip the glass into the rock salt. Add the simple syrup, tequila and triple sec to the shaker. Add ice and shake for 15 seconds. Strain and pour into glass. Enjoy your pesticide-free cocktail!

The term sulfite is shorthand for sulfur dioxide (SO_2), an inorganic salt used in wine and food because of its antioxidant and preservative properties. Used since 1664, sulfating agents are generally considered to be harmless when consumed, unless you are one of the unlucky 0.05% of the population who has a sulfite sensitivity. Any wine that contains more than 10 parts per million (ppm) of SO_2 must be labeled "contains sulfites." Even wine that does not contain added sulfites has sulfites in it, merely from the fact that it is a by-product of the fermentation process.

Any wine sold in the United States that contains added sulfites at a level over 100 ppm of SO_2 cannot be considered "organic," even if everything else about it is. Those wines must be labeled "made from organically grown grapes." I also found it interesting that the element molybdenum is necessary for the enzyme that breaks down sulfites. Well, perhaps my unusually high molybdenum levels were not a bad thing for drinking wines with added sulfites.

Knowing all this still didn't exactly answer the question of toxicity. I finally found some information on an organic wine website that stated, "Sulfite agents, when properly handled, are not intrinsically toxic to humans or to the environment, and many feel they are essential in order to prevent oxidation or bacterial spoilage. Therefore, American and European organic winemaking standards allow for the addition of strictly regulated amounts of SO_2."[2] Additional research I found stated that sulfiting agents are not teratogenic, mutagenic or carcinogenic in laboratory animals. In theory, unless you have sensitivity to sulfites or have asthma, it sounded like sulfites posed little risk of toxicity.

The final question about organic wines that I had was based on a statement I read in the paper a few weeks prior to looking for organic wines. And that was the claim that pesticides and other chemicals like herbicides used in conventional wine growing do not survive the fermentation process, thereby leaving few, if any, contaminants in the final product. I found this to be totally false. According to a 2008 study done by the Pesticide Action Network in Europe, pesticides were found in all 34 of the conventional wines they tested and a low level of pesticide residue in one of six organic wines. On average, each wine sampled contained more than 4 pesticides, with one bottle containing 10.[3]

Organic wines, with or without sulfites, were definitely the way to go. I certainly had no intention of drinking pesticides. The next time I went into our favorite grocery store, Ballard Market, I stopped to chat with the wine steward. Wine expert? Well, whatever you call the guy who manages the wine and beer in a grocery store. I had spoken with the wine-steward-expert guy in the past regarding biodynamic wines and his background working for a vineyard. He's a veritable wealth of knowledge on wine and, since I generally ask him things he likes talking about, he's usually quite helpful. I don't know what his actual name is, but his name tag says "Wayno," which I think might be some play on words for "wino" and "Wayne."

Prior to going to the store, I had done some online research on wines produced by a local winery called Snoqualmie Vineyards. They had a group of wines under the Naked label that are made with 100% organically produced grapes, even though they are not considered an organic wine since they have added sulfites. I knew they were sold in some of the Town and Country Markets of which Ballard Market was a member. I had just found the Snoqualmie Vineyards wines in the store when Wayno asked me if I needed any help. At that point I asked if they carried any of the Naked wines (they didn't). So I asked him what wines they did carry that were made from organically grown grapes but weren't certified as organic.

He was kind enough (and knowledgeable enough) to point out about six different wineries that used organically grown grapes. Since I was sick of the white wine I had been drinking, I picked up four bottles of reds. This is a bit much, but I figured I would get them while I remembered which ones were which. The wines made with organically grown grapes were intermixed with all the other wines and I doubted that I would remember them all, even though I did write them down. With the holidays coming up I figured they would get consumed and it would be nice to have some wine with dinner without worrying about how many pesticides I was drinking.

Heating oil headaches

When I went to school to pick up the kids one afternoon in early November, I met up with another mom whom I oftentimes chat with. She was complaining about a home-heating-oil leak that had occurred in her basement that morning. It was a result of switching over their heating fuel to natural gas and leaving the oil furnace as a backup. Somewhere along the way, the pipe with the heating oil leading to the furnace sprung a leak. It wasn't a huge leak, a cup or so of oil, but just enough to make the whole house noticeably stinky and necessary to call someone in to fix the problem.

This mom friend of mine, Io, had been exposed to the oil for a couple of hours and was complaining of headaches and dizziness. Since we have heating oil as our main source of home heating, I wondered how many of her symptoms were caused by the oil in her basement and how potentially toxic the exposure might be. We were certainly just as much at risk of exposure, however small, and it would be good to know upfront what the issues were.

After poking around briefly on the Internet, I found some basic information on heating oil spills from the Wisconsin Department of Health Services.[4] Before you even get to the meat of the information, there's a huge warning at the top of the web page: "Fuel oil is a hazardous substance. Respond immediately to fuel oil spills. Clean up small drips and spills by following the instructions in this fact sheet. For spills involving more than one gallon of fuel oil, hire a cleanup company specializing in hazardous materials and spill response." That was a little unsettling.

Aside from all the other inherent issues with a heating-oil spill in your home, the salient health issues can be summed up by the simple fact that fuel oil contains many substances that vary in their toxicity. Short-term exposure can cause headaches, nausea and dizziness, and prolonged exposure can cause serious health problems such as liver and kidney damage, increased blood pressure, other blood problems and cancer. Long-term exposure to benzene, the most toxic component of fuel oil, is known to cause leukemia.

This brought me to my next question — what kind of vapor or toxic fumes are released when we burn this stuff? According to the Lung Association of Canada, "the burning of fossil fuels such as coal, oil, natural gas or propane as well as biomass sources such as wood, all release chemicals into the air. These chemicals include sulphur oxides (SOx), nitrogen oxides (NOx), volatile organic compounds (VOCs), particulate matter (PM), carbon monoxide (CO) and other toxic material. These pollutants can have direct effects on respiratory and cardiovascular health."[5]

In essence, aside from geothermal power or electricity from hydro, solar or wind power, the fumes from any home-heating fuel are going to have some toxicity. Fortunately, most oil furnaces and the filters control many of the fumes and particulates produced. That is, assuming that you change them. I found that it was recommended that you change the furnace filter before heating season begins and again about halfway through. The last time we had had our oil furnace serviced was the previous Christmas, when we came home from vacation to a freezing house and realized that we had run out of heating oil while we were gone.

Thanks to an emergency oil delivery and servicing, we were quickly back up and running and out of 40 degree temperatures in the house. Since I wanted to minimize the amount of gunk being expelled from our oil furnace, I called the oil company and had someone come out for our annual tune-up and filter change. I hoped this would keep the toxic emissions as low as possible short of not using it at all.

Because we were in the midst of my blog's Freeze Yer Buns Challenge, with the thermostat set at 62°F during the day and 55°F at night, the central heat from our oil furnace really hadn't been coming on too frequently yet. Between the space heater, which runs on the electricity we get from wind and hydro, and ambient air temperatures outside being somewhat warm in early November coupled with passive solar heating, our fuel consumption at the start of the challenge was minimal. The central oil-based heat only went on briefly in the morning and again in the evening if things were too chilly. Usually the heat from the kitchen kept the rest of the living spaces warm so it was really morning time when the furnace got some use. In any case, exposure to the heating oil and the emissions from burning it was low at the early stages of the project.

Teflon slip-up

While I was out meeting a friend for coffee one Saturday morning, my husband was surreptitiously baking a cake. Before I left to hang out with a new friend, Kathy (the co-owner of the Salish Sea Trading Cooperative — our sailboat vegetable delivery service), Hank had asked me what kind of dessert I wanted him to bake that weekend. My answer was "none" because I had recently weighed myself and, between a three-week summer trip and his weekly baked goods, I was horrified to see that I had put on even more weight. I was officially 20 pounds overweight and was determined to lean up a little bit before I started doing any more TV filming.

Two nights before my coffee date I had met up with the producer of a television show that I had worked on the previous year. It was a green makeover-style show where a group of consultants (and cast members) would analyze a family's lifestyle and give them suggestions on how to green their life and reduce their carbon footprint. If the family met the challenges we proposed to them, they would win some sort of gift. In the case of the pilot, the family won a landscaping makeover complete with raised beds for growing vegetables.

The pilot episode was a riot to film — none of us had done anything like it before. The cast members had done some promotional work on the final clip and then did a big blow-out premiere in Seattle, which was one of the highlights of filming and something I'll never forget. The people I worked with were truly a joy and I am happy to call them all new friends. In any case, the move from filming the pilot episode to finding a network to pick up the show had stalled out. When I met with the producer, Rose Thornton, I suggested bringing shorter snippets of content to the Web to help build a fan base and keep bringing people back for more. The idea was to film segments less than 10 minutes long on sustainable topics to be hosted on YouTube with an occasional family makeover thrown in for good measure.

As a result, that weekend one of the things on my mind was that, if I was going to be filming again, I should at least get back in shape. I had already started walking 30 minutes in the morning after dropping the kids off at school, but I needed to be more careful about what I was eating as my weight had continued to slowly go up. So, when the dessert question came up, all I could think about was slowing down on the intake. It sounds horribly vain but the camera does add more pounds than you'd think.

When I came back home to find that Hank was in the middle of baking a cake, I didn't think twice about it. I just figured I'd try to show some restraint. Although I must say that working from home, alone, with a cake staring at you every day when you are too busy to make lunch makes it awfully tempting to indulge. It wasn't until he had taken the cake out of the oven that I noticed he had used one of our remaining Teflon cake pans. Since it was a Bundt cake with fancy edging, you really can't get away too easily without nonstick and there aren't too many options for alternatives. Even Fat Daddio's Bundt pans were all nonstick pans. I think Hank had completely forgotten about the Teflon issue and was just blithely baking away.

The next day, when I went food shopping (and hanging out with Wayno), I picked up a few locally made, fair trade organic dark chocolate bars to prevent me from eating the Teflon cake without feeling too deprived. Later that night, when my guard was down and I had completely forgotten about the Teflon *and* the chocolate bars, I had a small piece of cake. Just a small piece of nonstick, though. Later in the week I made sure that I didn't slip up again and avoided the cake like the plague. I also made double sure that I didn't slip up again and absentmindedly use the rice cooker (it has a nonstick coating). I brushed the dust off my brain and made rice the old-fashioned way—on the stove. I figured that made up for the tiny piece of cake, but really that Teflon cake still counted. I promptly put the rice cooker out to pasture to prevent anything similar from happening again.

A few days later it was Veterans Day and we all were home—the kids from school and my husband from work. I had been talking to a friend at the kids' school about what their plans were for the holiday and he mentioned that his wife was going to make breakfast for everyone. After I told Hank about their plans for the day, he decided he wanted to make waffles for breakfast. Usually, during the school week, it's a mad rush to get everyone out the door and we're lucky if the kids are wearing clothes let alone enjoying a hot breakfast. So, it was nice to have a relaxed day during the week to spend some extra time at the table.

Henry, of course, didn't want waffles as he has his food comfort rules he has to stick to (food anxiety and OCD stuff), but Emma was game. She had been battling a little virus and hadn't eaten dinner the night before so she was starving by the time the waffles started coming. I generally don't like eating much for breakfast and I'm not particularly fond of waffles, but I decided I should join in the fun and had one. It wasn't until later in the day that I realized that our waffle iron has a nonstick coating. These nonstick coatings are on so many kitchen products that it's hard to keep track of them. I had completely forgotten this one since we don't use it very often. That week ended up being a big Teflon failure.

Getting clean with grease

I didn't realize you could actually make your own bar soap until I saw the movie *Fight Club* about 10 years ago. Granted, I wasn't planning on making my own soap from rendered liposuction waste and Draino, but the whole concept was completely eye-opening for me. All it takes to make soap is a few simple ingredients—water, lye and fat—the very same ingredients that have been used since the time of the Ancient Romans to clean bodies as well as clothes. Yet, throughout history, Westerners have had an on-again, off-again relationship with personal cleanliness and it really wasn't until the late 1800s that soap became cheap enough that the middle class could afford it. Up until that time, soap was mainly used only for washing clothes and floors. Since the 1920s, Americans have been inundated with advertisements for products geared toward keeping us clean. And since then, our frequency of bathing has increased substantially. You no longer hear deodorant commercials touting the fact that "you can even skip a day" because the most recent assumption when it comes to personal grooming is that you are bathing daily.

I think that, like most consumers, I got so used to buying products (most of which contain dozens of unpronounceable ingredients) off the shelf that I didn't even question what they were made out of, or, more importantly, if I could even make them myself. Generally, few of us have a closet full of chemicals we could use to mimic our favorite petroleum-based bar soaps and body washes, but a bar soap made with natural fats, water, lye and some essential oils? That's something I could easily get into.

Soon after seeing that movie so many years ago, I purchased a few soap-making books and embarked on making my own bath soap. I liked the fact that I had total control over the ingredients going into my homemade soap and could make it entirely vegetarian by using my favorite oils like coconut oil, cocoa butter, avocado oil and olive oil. Or I could cater it to skin type, custom-making goat-milk soap bars to give to my brother for his eczema or coffee-ground soap to help clean up dirty hands in the kitchen. It didn't matter what kind of soap I was making, I was hooked.

Over the intervening years, I haven't made as much of my own soap as I'd like to, mostly because it does take a bit of work and patience and, with small children in the house, you have to be careful to do it when they aren't around because of the danger when dealing with caustic lye. Most importantly, however, I stopped making my own soap because, since I knew what ingredients went into high-quality bar soap, I could easily identify off-the-shelf soaps that were similar to what I could make at home but without the work, the waiting time for the bars to cure and the fumes.

The manufacturing of soap had pretty much remained the same from ancient times until around 1916 when a shortage of soap-making fats during World War I precipitated the use of synthetic detergents, the sales of which had surpassed the sale of soap by 1953. These detergents, used alone or in combination with fat- and sodium hydroxide (lye)–based soaps, are most often found in modern soap bars used for personal cleansing.[6] The problem is that the detergents aren't all that great for your skin and can

---

Lavender Goat Milk Soap

Ingredients (makes 4 lb.)
- 6.5 oz. lye (sodium hydroxide)
- 16 oz. whole goat milk (cold)
- 17 oz. olive oil
- 17 oz. coconut oil
- 8 oz. palm oil
- 2–3 oz. lavender essential oil

Directions
Wearing safety goggles and rubber gloves, add the lye to the goat milk, stirring the mixture to combine completely. Set the goat milk and lye mixture aside and let it cool to between 100°F and 125°F.

Combine the oils and heat them to 100°F–125°F. When both the lye mixture and oil mixture are in the proper temperature range, combine. Use precautions to avoid splashing (you can use vinegar to neutralize the soap mixture for cleanup).

Stir the mixture until it thickens and traces (where you can see the soap leave a "trace" when spooned across the surface). Once the mixture is at trace, add your essential oil, incorporate it into the soap and then pour the thickened liquid into your soap molds.

When the soap is hard enough to remove (but still soft enough to cut), remove the soap from your molds, cut as needed and let cure for 4 weeks, preferably covered with a towel.

---

end up being skin irritants. More importantly, the vast majority of these soaps contain synthetic fragrance (parfum), which potentially harbors phthalates.

Up until this project, I hadn't used a bar of conventional soap in years, with the exception of the previous summer when we were on vacation and I used some Dove Sensitive Skin soap which, in actuality, reads like a laundry list of chemical ingredients. In many cases when we travel we take our own soap but we have also been fortunate that many hotels tend to carry the gourmet version of soap, which means they supply soaps that are made with natural ingredients. In other words, the kind of soap that makes you feel like you are being pampered by the hotel — something like a lavender goat milk soap.

Bodywash brainwash

Bodywash has been marketed to female consumers since the mid-1980s and recently there has been a huge push in advertising for more manly body wash products to get male consumers equally hooked. Between "ribbons of moisture," bath poufs and men's showering "tools," bodywash as a product has been an enormous success. When asked, many people have very strong opinions in the bar soap versus bodywash debate. As a result, sales of bar soap are slipping and the consequences extend to more than just cost and convenience.[7] In 2008, the market research firm Mintel reported that 29% of women said they never buy bar soap, compared with 24% of men.[8] Those statistics are changing as men's bodywash sales increase. Many of the men's bodywash products are being touted as multipurpose products doing double duty as both a bodywash and a shampoo. Some companies advertise their bodywash as also a shampoo and shave gel.

Clever advertising geared toward women, who purchase over 80% of the products in a household, has also increased the switch from bar soap to bodywash for men.[9] The bodywash market went from $480 million in 2003 to $733 million in 2008, an increase of 53%. According to Mintel's projections, revenue will top $1 billion in 2013. Data from Nielsen, another market research company, shows that men's formulas are growing more rapidly than women's and unisex products, from a 17% share of overall category revenue in 2005 to 28% in 2009.[10]

The underlying issues with bodywash aren't just the ingredients found in all those plastic squeeze bottles. To start, the average person goes through about 200 bottles of bodywash in their lifetime.[11] All the extra plastic packaging and plastic scrubbers that are sold or purchased along with the bodywash have a limited lifetime and get thrown away or, if recyclable, get downcycled at best. The environmental impact of the chemicals used in bodywash is not inconsequential either and some estimate that it takes more than 800 years for those chemicals to disappear from our water systems. However, with a steadily increasing stream of these products entering our waterways each day, "disappearing" seems like an impossible task. Compared to bar soap, liquid bodywash has even more of a potential for hazardous toxins. In order to make the soap liquid, manufacturers rely heavily on petroleum-based cleansers, focusing particularly on sodium lauryl and laureth sulfates, as well as other chemicals.

I, personally, don't use bodywash and really haven't over the years, mostly because I prefer the ease of using a bar soap and, more importantly, I am extremely sensitive to the strong fragrances contained in most bodywashes. In addition, I don't like all the plastic waste, however recyclable the containers are. There are more "natural" bodywashes now available on the market, but since I've never caught onto the bodywash craze, my aversion to the plastic waste trumps anything available. My husband doesn't like them either and, because we just don't buy it, the kids don't use liquid body soap. The Dr. Bronner's organic bar soap we have used for years continued to be perfect for this project.

Deodorant part deux

It was official—I stunk. I loved my homemade deodorant but it didn't love me. It worked better than anything else I was using and it didn't contain any aluminum of any sort. It also didn't have any parabens, preservatives or artificial fragrances — nothing. Even lacking all that, though, it left me smelling great. The only problem with it was that it irritated the hell out of my armpits. I thought that reducing the concentration of baking soda (as a total percentage) would improve things but I still found it to be gritty and, after a while, it left my armpits red and irritated.

Since the irritation began, I had switched back to using the Rock (aka Crystal deodorant) full-time, trying the Crystal deodorant in both liquid and solid forms. My brother and husband swear that the solid version works better but I feel like I'm just rubbing a wet piece of glass on my armpits with about the same results. By the early afternoon, especially after going walking in the morning after dropping the kids off at school, I smelled of B.O. The liquid Crystal worked a little better for me, keeping the stink bomb surprise until a little later so I didn't reek until closer to dinnertime. With my homemade stuff, I didn't stink at all. No B.O. stench. Just red, unhappy pits.

I had used the Ban Roll-On Unscented (the one that ranked a 1 out of 10 on the EWG database) once since the beginning of this project and only because I was being filmed for a television segment for the local news. These situations always make me nervous and I figured worrying about giant, wet pit stains wasn't going to help matters much. For some reason, the week after filming the segment I had an ad pop up on my Gmail account suggesting a clinical deodorant that was supposed to really help.

Apparently Google was reading my mind. Or could smell my armpits through my laptop. I don't know why I clicked on the link, but I was curious as to how potentially toxic a super-antiperspirant would be. I checked out the ingredients and mostly it was more of an issue with the fragrances (and potential phthalates) in it. This led me to look into the product Certain Dri Antiperspirant Roll-On, which is another clinical-strength antiperspirant. I plugged it into the EWG Cosmetic Database and was surprised to learn that it only ranked a 1, just like the unscented Ban.[12] Since it contains so few ingredients, it made some sense. The only real ingredient at issue was the aluminum chloride, which is the ingredient that stops the sweating.

Since I would be doing more and more filming for a variety of projects I was working on, I made a mental note to pick up some Certain Dri for those occasions. In the meantime, I spent some time completely reworking my homemade deodorant. I made a new batch that removed all the baking soda since that seemed to be the element causing the problem. I figured if that worked out I could add a little baking soda at a time to find out what my skin sensitivity threshold was.

Squeaky clean

When I was a teenager, I started using one cleanser to wash my face and another for the rest of my body. I was told early on that soap was too harsh and too drying, stripping your fragile facial skin of moisture. Of course, since I was using petroleum-based soaps back then, it certainly seemed true. My skin always felt extremely tight after washing my face with soap, whether it was bar soap or liquid soap. In my mid-teens I did some modeling and I was admonished by my agent never to use bar soap. It was recommended that I use Noxzema to wash my face.

Back then, I was prone to the occasional acne breakout, and using Noxzema helped clear up my skin. I dutifully used this product for years until I eventually switched over to some of the newer facial cleansers that were coming on the market. I then hopped over to a version of Neutrogena's Clean and Clear, dabbling in department-store brand facial cleansers (my favorite was Estée Lauder's Perfectly Clean Splash Away Foaming Cleanser) and finally settling on a natural brand. I thought I had eliminated the nasty chemicals in my facial cleanser by using a natural one, Alba Pineapple Enzyme Facial Cleanser. But I was wrong.

The ubiquity of advertising for facial cleansers in women's magazines and on television proves, to some degree, that I am not the only one convinced that in order to have a clean, healthy face, you need a special product. Was my facial skin really that delicate and did the pH really need to be maintained by fancy products? Do products like Neutrogena Deep Cleanser really "remove the toxins" as they claim in their latest ads and, furthermore, what toxins are you putting on your skin instead? I was extremely wary of using anything besides a facial cleanser on my face, because I had been so well trained by advertising and the whole allure of the beauty-product industry. When I read on a few blogs that some people were switching back to using natural bar soap on their faces, I thought they didn't have the same oily/dry combination skin that was prone to acne and so could get away with it. However, for the sake of reducing my exposure to chemicals and to reduce the amount of plastics I was consuming, I bit the bullet and tried washing my face with my favorite Dr. Bronner's bar soap.

To say I was a little nervous was an understatement. I was very fearful that I would have a huge acne breakout and that my skin would experience massive dryness and rapid aging. It all sounds overly dramatic, but that was what was running through my head the first time I washed my face in the shower with natural bar soap. As it turned out, my face didn't rot off. I didn't break out and I didn't experience progeria, or any other accelerated aging disease. In fact, my skin felt fine – just as good as it did with the $20 Estée Lauder cleanser. But did it deliver a "deliciously refreshing foam [that] gently yet thoroughly cleans and rebalances skin"? Did it "splash away with no soapy film, no trace of impurities"? I don't know about the deliciously refreshing foam part (except for when I used the peppermint soap bar), but Dr. Bronner's easily met all the department-store brand's claims of clean, rebalanced, impurity-free skin. All toxin-free, for that matter.

For the purposes of this book and, even before getting tested for phthalates and parabens, I just couldn't bring myself to use anything else on my face besides Dr. Bronner's. I considered using Dove or some other more mainstream soap or even the old Alba product I still had hanging around in the closet. But I just couldn't do it. I could muster up the courage to put some chemical-laden soap on the rest of my body, but I just wasn't able to put it on my face. This really doesn't make sense because I was using a chemical soup of sunblock on my face during the same time period. Maybe I was starting to develop early signs of toxiphobia.

Going zits up

When my husband's immune system was initially suppressed due to his cancer, he started experiencing more issues with skin infections. Around the same time, I started having similar problems myself. I don't know how related they are, but I started getting skin infections on my legs where I shaved and began using an acne cleanser to help clear things up. I had picked up some Neutrogena Body Clear Body Wash and had been using it for quite some time. I really didn't want to look too closely at the ingredient list because I knew that there were some not-so-nice chemical customers hiding in there and it was working for me. I was having a lot fewer problems with ingrown hairs and skin infections and, ultimately, ignorance was very blissful.

Alas, look closely I finally did and I was not too happy with what I saw. Salicylic acid was the primary active ingredient but there were also some familiar unsavory chemicals as well as the chemical triclosan, which is an antibacterial and is considered a pesticide by the EPA. Another very popular acne cleanser is Murad Acne Body Wash and it too contains some chemical ingredients to avoid.[13] So, to avoid all the chemicals, I tried the natural-sounding Nature's Gate Corrective Cleansing Treatment and was rather pleased with it—until I looked a little closer at the full ingredient listing. Initially, I thought it only had salicylic acid in it as its main active ingredient but, upon closer inspection, I found it also contained a few other similar chemicals. Unfortunately, the sample I was using also contained triclosan, although it looks like it has been removed from more recent formulations. The biggest drawback to this product was that it is nearly impossible to find in stores and it contained some ingredients that I didn't want to use, even without the triclosan. It seemed to be doing a decent job and had less potentially toxic ingredients than the Neutrogena product I was using, but since I would have to order it online, all these facts conspired against my using it.

I was having a hell of a time trying to find a natural product that didn't have potential toxins in it. One of these so-called natural products (by Hyland's) even had resorcinol in it, which ranks a 10 on the Skin Deep database.[14] I searched high and low for a product that didn't contain anything I didn't want to put on my skin and ended up making my own homemade natural acne body wash, which relied on essential oils for antiseptic and antibacterial properties.

Homemade Acne Wash

Ingredients

- 0.5–1 tsp essential oils (see below for suggestions)
- 2 cups unscented liquid soap (like Dr. Bronner's)
- Aspirin (if desired*)

Directions

Add one or more essential oils to the liquid soap. Mix well, store in a bottle and use in place of your regular acne body wash.

*If you want something stronger and need to add in something similar to salicylic acid, dissolve 5 uncoated aspirin in a small amount of water and mix into the liquid soap. Acetylsalicylic acid (aka aspirin) ranks #7 on the Skin Deep database, so use with care.

Lavender essential oil is well known as an antiseptic and an antibacterial. Lavender oil is also used to combat acne, eczema and seborrhea. It is excellent when used as a preventative acne treatment that effectively stops future breakouts while clearing the redness often associated with acne-prone skin.

Tea tree oil is another excellent antibacterial treatment, making it a great acne fighter as well as a general-purpose wound cleaner. It has been proven effective in killing bacteria when applied topically. As an acne treatment, tea tree oil is fast-acting and acts to clear up the skin while calming the affected area.

Eucalyptus essential oil is very effective at clearing up blackheads, pimples and blemishes on the skin.

Yellow gold

After a while I gave up on using the homemade acne wash because I found something else that has been incredibly effective. And it had to do with researching my husband's cancer and looking at more natural supplements and other nonpharmaceutical approaches to cancer. I am in no way convinced of the movement *against* Western medicine when it comes to cancer treatments. I know a number of people, family members included, who definitely wouldn't still be alive if it weren't for Western cancer treatments. However, I am also not against seeing what else is out there as far as diet and nutrition go for making a cancer patient more receptive to treatment and helping their immune system identify and, essentially, "mop up" cancer cells.

One treatment that had been getting a bit of research in the fight against multiple myeloma was the use of curcumin, otherwise known as turmeric, a yellow spice used mostly notably in Indian cuisine. Studies have shown an anticancer effect in various phases of cancer development, growth and proliferation. Studies done at the M. D. Anderson Cancer Research Center in Houston, Texas, showed this effect on a variety of cancer cells including prostate and breast tumor cell lines. And studies also showed that, when curcumin was added to human cells with myeloma, the curcumin stopped the cells from replicating and the remaining cells died.[15]

Turmeric is also well known as an anti-inflammatory, as a guard against multiple sclerosis and Alzheimer's and as an aid in wound healing. That was enough for me to start trying it out as a supplement. My husband wanted to talk to his oncologist first before starting to take it on his own as he might gain some insight into therapeutic levels or find out his impression on the efficacy of oral treatment. Since turmeric also acts as a blood thinner and since my husband is on blood thinner medication (because of his chemo), I didn't want there to be any complications from taking it. For me, however, I got some just to see if it helped with the skin infections.

Much to my surprise, I stopped having the dreaded skin infections, even without using the acne soap. The form of turmeric that I was using was somewhat expensive since I bought a local, organic version, but all costs aside, it was still cheaper than the alternative. I had also read that Indians traditionally used turmeric for skin infections as a topical treatment, so when I had a particularly annoying bump, a straight application mixed in coconut oil cleared it up almost overnight.

Makeup!

Trying to find makeup that doesn't contain questionable ingredients has gotten easier over the last few years but, for the most part, it is still considerably difficult. Even those products on the market that claim they are organic can still be chock-full of artificial fragrances and parabens. Months before writing this book I had invested in a variety of cosmetics from a drugstore organics line. I was very excited that a drugstore brand of makeup was carrying an organic line, sporting recyclable packaging and products in bamboo. I didn't look too closely at the ingredients because they were organic, which meant they were good for you, right? At that point I was more concerned with how they compared to my usual repertoire of Estée Lauder, MAC, Maybelline and Cover Girl cosmetics. Not only did the organic line not work as well, but they also still had a lot of chemical junk in them.

I then went on a search for cosmetics that truly didn't have anything nasty in them. The next time I was at our natural food co-op I saw that they carried a couple lines of makeup that were locally manufactured, Gabriel Cosmetics and Zuzu Luxe (also owned by Gabriel). I wrote down the names of the brands to look up the ingredients online and really liked what I saw. I found out that the products from Gabriel Cosmetics makeup had few unnerving ingredients and those that were considered questionable were mostly things like mica or retinol (Vitamin A). After purchasing a few different things from both lines, I found that their products worked nearly as well as my old, conventional makeup. Because the ingredients are natural, they don't go on as smoothly, but they were close enough. The eyeliner will never compare to my MAC eyeliner and the mascara rubs off way too easily, but all in all, it made for a satisfactory substitute.

I looked into a lot of mineral makeup lines on the market, many of which are also very good, but some contained questionable ingredients so you really have to look at their listings to make sure they aren't riding the "minerals" wave. I know there are other brands out there with few or no toxins in them (like Josie Maran Cosmetics), but they aren't as easily accessible for me and I'm fairly satisfied with what I have. I wouldn't mind finding a better eyeliner or mascara but I generally don't wear much makeup so it wasn't a huge priority.

Lubed and lotioned

I had been using the Alba body lotion (with all its parabens and whatnot) as mentioned before for years, but had also started using a different product that didn't contain anything nasty in it. Hugo Naturals Vanilla Sweet Orange Body Lotion is a product that we had used for about a year as a hand lotion, and I knew that it was mild enough to use all over, even on my face. Not only does it smell fantastic, it isn't greasy and is absorbed quickly. I can't stand moisturizers in general because I don't like feeling as if I'm coated in a layer of Crisco. This is a problem with many of the "natural" moisturizers available on the market because they tend to use heavier oils. Coconut oil (and a few others) is an exception, however. I have successfully used coconut oil on my face as both a makeup remover and a moisturizer for several years and have never had any skin problems or breakouts. Coconut oil does a fantastic job of keeping my skin hydrated and, more importantly, is absorbed relatively quickly.

I decided about 10 years previous to this project that I should probably start really taking care of my facial skin to help ward off signs of premature aging. I dutifully began a regimen of department-store brand cleansers, moisturizers, eye creams, anti-aging lotions, sunscreens and scrubs. I was around 30 at the time and I figured that this head start would help me out tremendously and I'd be looking as fresh as a daisy well into my 60s. Nowadays, it doesn't sound so extraordinary that a woman in her 30s would begin an anti-aging routine, but I thought I was ahead of the mark back then. And now it's not unusual for anti-aging products to be targeted at women in their 20s. Walmart's geoGirl line of cosmetics is marketed to girls aged 8–12, with a few anti-aging components thrown in for good measure. This particular product line is purportedly free of chemicals like parabens, phthalates and sulfates, with a minimal use of synthetic colors and fragrances, so it has that going for it at least.

In any case, during the decade I had been using these I had dropped some of the products and really just stuck with moisturizers, anti-aging lotions and microdermabrasion-type products with a healthy dollop of sunscreen. I mostly stuck with Estée Lauder products and even branched out to the *über*-expensive La Mer for a while, which was quite lovely but not really worth the cost. Over the last three years I had noticed a considerable aging of the skin around my eyes with a lot more dark circles, which I attributed to the immense amount of stress in my life. At that point, I quit some of the anti-aging products and started using a retinol-based product on the areas that were showing more wear and tear. I have to admit, I saw some extremely amazing results — my skin looked *years* younger. But I still saw wrinkles around my eyes that weren't there before and just chalked it up to aging.

Then, about a year ago, a few things happened. I started having an allergic reaction to an anti-aging product that I had received for review from Mad Hippie Skin Care and the retinol product really aggravated the skin around my eyes. It took a month of trying various products with no relief before I decided to start over. For a few months I stopped all commercial facial moisturizers cold turkey and switched entirely to a non-toxic product to solve the problems I was having. This meant that I was relying solely on coconut oil as my moisturizer. I used the coconut oil morning and night as an all-over facial moisturizer, applying it particularly heavily around my eyes. During that time I noticed two things. The first was that the circles under my eyes had lessened quite a bit. I chalked this up to less irritation and probable allergic reaction to the chemicals I had been exposing my facial skin to over the years. It certainly wasn't because I was getting more sleep. The second thing I noticed, and I honestly couldn't really believe this myself, was that the wrinkles around my eyes had all but disappeared.

It took me a while to figure out what the story was, but my theory was that my skin was recovering from the chemical and allergen burden. The coconut oil was providing enough moisture and plumping to make the wrinkles that I did have less visible. And, finally, from what I had been reading, coconut oil helps in preventing premature aging and degenerative diseases due to its antioxidant properties. Just using the coconut oil allowed my skin to fully recover and I was no longer feeling any irritation and burning like I was before I quit all the other products on my skin besides soap. Since then (and up to the point of getting my initial body burden tests done), I had gone back to using some of my old products, just for the purpose of this project and the testing. The facial moisturizer I was using was either sunscreen or an old Estée Lauder moisturizer of unknown ingredients. I didn't want to have another skin reaction by using the retinol product and, in any case, I had gotten rid of that product a while ago.

After getting the body burden testing done, I started using the Hugo Naturals body lotion product sometimes as a facial moisturizer in addition to the coconut oil. I also needed a daytime face cream that had a sunscreen in it for days when the sun actually did come out. It was less of a problem in November in Seattle, when gray skies are in abundance, but it was still important. There are several issues with many different chemical types of sunscreens, but suffice it to say for now that I wanted something with zinc oxide as a sunblock. And, just as important, I wanted one where the zinc oxide particles weren't nano-sized. (I'll cover all the nitty-gritty about sunscreens later.)

Of course, this day cream would also have to fit all the other criteria for natural ingredients but miraculously, after a bit of searching, I managed to find my holy grail of facial moisturizers. It was expensive and a little greasier than I was used to, but it worked really well and was absorbed quickly. The product, SanRe Supple Sunshine moisturizer, had an SPF 30 from zinc oxide, smelled good (a mix of rosemary and lavender) and didn't contain anything nasty, including any dreaded nano particles. In fact, even though it wouldn't taste very good, I'm pretty sure I could eat this day cream without any problems. Although the container was relatively small, it lasted a long time and I added it to my list of products that I would continue using long after this book project ended.

Another thing I was feeling like I was missing was something a little creamier to use as a moisturizer when I didn't need a sunblock, like at night. While I loved the coconut oil and still use it on my face twice a day around my eyes and for dry spots, it's a pain to apply, especially during the colder months when it's hard and you have to wait for it to melt from your body heat which, if you are also cold, takes a while.

I ran across the skincare line by Gabriel Cosmetics at my local Whole Foods and was ecstatic because I loved his cosmetics and trusted this line of products to not have a load of chemicals in them. I zeroed in on the Marine Anti-Aging Cream that contained blue-green algae and rosehip seed oil for increasing moisture and oxygen in my skin, and Vitamins A, C and E as proven age-fighting antioxidants. Again, this product had no scary ingredients and, although I wouldn't say this one was edible, it was about as natural as they come.

I didn't exactly have my hopes up for how it would perform as an anti-aging product since I figured it just couldn't compare to the chemical ones on the market. At the very least, it smelled good and felt good. It was too soon to tell whether or not it was doing anything, but I had high hopes for that furrow that was growing between my eyebrows.

Blocking out the sun

Since this project was going on during the months in Seattle where we rarely, if ever, see the sun, it is difficult to squeeze in the conversation about full-on sunscreen or sunblock because I wasn't using any, except for the SanRe product on my face. The rest of my body was hidden under clothing and we didn't take any tropical trips. Months earlier I had done some research on the ingredients in the sunblocks we had hanging around in the cabinets. Preventing skin cancer is very important to me, especially because I freckle very easily and I already see lots of moles and freckles developing on my kids. My abundance of moles and whatnot is more genetic than sun exposure–related, but I wanted to make sure that we were as protected as possible. Since my husband has serious sun sensitivity due to a number of medications he takes as well as immune system complications post-transplant (graft versus host disease of his skin), he needed to be protected even more than the rest of us. He also has allergic reactions to many of the chemical sunscreens out there, so trying to find something that fit all our needs *and* was as non-toxic as possible seemed almost impossible.

There are many issues with some of the sun protection products on the market, particularly the ones that get absorbed into the skin (chemical sunscreens) versus the kinds that sit on the skin (mineral sunscreens). When I looked at the ingredients in the eight or so different sunscreens we had in the house, they all had artificial fragrance and parabens in them. Not only that, but most of them also contained a mix of chemical sunscreens and other problematic ingredients. One of those bonus ingredients is Vitamin A, or retinyl palmitate. Studies have shown that, when applied to the skin in the presence of sunlight, retinyl palmitate may speed up the development of skin tumors and lesions. Another big ingredient no-no I found in many of our products was the chemical sunscreen oxybenzone, which is a notorious hormone disruptor. In fact, scientists have called for parents to avoid using oxybenzone on children due to penetration and toxicity concerns.[16]

Mineral blocking agents are the best bet when choosing a non-toxic sunscreen. These sit on the skin, instead of being absorbed into the body, and also effectively block UVA light. I can't say I love the chalky effect of some of the mineral sunscreens, though. The nano or micronized mineral sunscreens get around that by making the particles small enough to be slightly absorbed to avoid the Casper the Friendly Ghost look. However, no FDA studies have been done on the absorption of nanoparticles and their health effects and no studies have been done on damaged or fragile skin to show how the particles may or may not penetrate the skin and end up elsewhere in your system.[17] Frankly, using nanoparticles just wasn't worth the potential risk.

The Environmental Working Group puts out an annual list of the best sunscreens and their relative risk. From that list, I selected Badger Sunscreen for Face and Body, SPF 30, as our sunblock of choice. It is zinc oxide–based with particles greater than 100 nm. The rest of the ingredients are harmless. I can't say it's my favorite sunblock—that award goes to the products with the chemical agents. If the mineral sunscreen ends up being too much of a pain to rub in and we are less likely to use it because of that, the chemical sunscreen of choice would contain avobenzone and preferably no fragrance or parabens. Assuming, that is, one exists.

The best thing, of course, is to practice avoidance during daylight hours when the sun is strongest. When our family spends any time at the beach or in the pool, all of us wear rash guards for sun protection in addition to sunscreen. My husband and I always wear long-sleeved rash guards. The kids wear short-sleeved ones. I generally will wear longer surfing-style shorts at the beach as well. I can't say I'm looking too sexy poolside but it's really not what I'm aiming for anyway. I want to have fun and not get burned in the process. Large hats are also something we employ when out in the sun. This isn't realistic when you are in the water, but for all other times we try to wear hats. It's a little harder to get the kids to comply on this one detail, so we load them up with sunscreen and keep exposure times low.

'Poos and don'ts

I already mentioned my ill-fated attempt at trying the "no-poo" method of washing my hair with baking soda and water. Over the years, I've also tried numerous other so-called natural alternatives to commercial shampoo. I've tried Giovanni Tea Tree Triple Treat Invigorating Shampoo, which was more than just invigorating, it was painful. I found it to be so minty and tingly it felt like my skin was on fire. Not on my scalp, but on my face and other areas it touched. The product ended up making my hair so dried out it looked like straw. Even though it was certified organic and didn't contain any lauryl/laureth sulfates, I didn't like it one bit.

I've also tried shampoos like Burt's Bees Very Volumizing Pomegranate Shampoo. It doesn't contain any sodium lauryl sulfite (SLS) ingredients and it shows. It smelled great, but the lather was less than impressive and I couldn't stand using it for more than a few days. It didn't feel like it cleaned my hair and it, too, left my hair dried out. I always ended up going back to my regular, chemical-laden shampoo. Clearly, the Biolage Shampoo and Conditioner I was using (high in parabens and other nasties), although fantastic at cleaning and conditioning, wasn't going to meet my non-toxic standards. Even the Aveda haircare products I have used off and on for years still had some questionable ingredients. While Aveda has made some strides in removing parabens from their products, there are other things in there that I didn't trust.

I had been using Aveda's Smooth Infusion Shampoo, which I really liked. Unfortunately, it contained sulfates, which are harsh on skin and hair and the jury is still out on their health effects. It also contained fragrance (parfum), which could potentially contain phthalates, although they claim it is plant derived. It contained limonene, which ranks a 6 on the cosmetic safety database, as well as linalool, which ranks a 5. Needless to say, this product wasn't a clear yes or no, but in the end I stopped using it because of my unanswered questions about some of the ingredients.

My other alternatives were to continue using the shampoo bars and/or find an off-the-shelf product that was organic and non-toxic—and actually worked. I liked the shampoo bars, but we had run out of the homemade bars and sometimes the Camamu brand of shampoo bars that we liked was hard to find in our stores. I had heard some really good things about the John Masters Organic line of haircare products so I went in search of some conditioner while I was using the rest of the bars.

I found the John Masters line of products at Whole Foods and started off with a thick conditioner. It wasn't as good as I was used to from Biolage and Aveda, but it did the job. Because this product doesn't contain a heavy dollop of dimethicones and other silicones, it just can't compare, but the ingredients in the John Masters Lavender & Avocado Intensive Conditioner were relatively inert. There wasn't a scary ingredient to be found in there. After having success with the conditioner, I bit the bullet and sprang for the shampoo. Again, the ingredients in the John Masters Lavender Rosemary Shampoo were as clean as a whistle. The most potentially offensive ingredient was yarrow extract (according to the Cosmetic Database). Yarrow is a flowering plant and can cause allergies, which wasn't an issue for me.

More importantly, these mostly organic products didn't just contain non-toxic ingredients, they actually worked. Did they work as well as the Biolage and Aveda products? No, I would have to argue that they did not. You just can't compare them to detergent-based products. But then again, it's their toxic ingredients that make them work—and at what cost? And speaking of cost, many would argue that John Masters is expensive, but it's really not much more than I was already paying for my other products. If cost were more of an issue for me, I would stick to shampoo bars and coconut oil for deep conditioning. Once I got the shampoo and conditioner replacements under control I started working on the styling products, which was much more of a challenge.

Goops and greases

Months before, when I started doing research for this book and started seeing all the horrors and high cancer risks of many of the ingredients we were slathering daily on our bodies, I decided to take a peek at the ingredients in the hairstyling product my husband used. I was more concerned about his body's ability to handle all these potentially toxic ingredients because of his cancer, his compromised immune system and his susceptibility to cancer cell proliferation. If an ingredient was suspected of being a carcinogen, then he really didn't need it taxing his immune system and I didn't want him being exposed to it.

Many companies and individuals representing the chemical industry argue that small doses of potential toxins like parabens and phthalates and polyethylene glycols (PEGs) don't hurt the human body, that we are capable of processing them and ridding them from our systems. That is true to some degree, but given the fact that there are so many products that contain a maelstrom of chemical ingredients, with some estimates that the average American uses upward of 10 products a day, it begins to add up. And your body has to work that much harder to "process" all those chemicals. With multiple parabens and phthalates in each product, sometimes applied multiple times a day, your body is working full-time to eliminate them. And then those small doses aren't negligible anymore.

In my husband's case, he had stopped using traditional shaving cream years ago, opting instead for a shaving brush and a natural shaving bar soap. That was non-toxic so I wasn't worried about that. Post-stem cell transplant his skin was more sensitive and he started using an aftershave lotion. I made sure that I picked it out for him and the most readily available one with the least number of chemicals in it was Burt's Bees Natural Skin Care Aftershave which claims it is 100% natural. I couldn't find anything suspicious in it. A while back I also made sure he stopped using traditional shampoo and had been getting alternatives for him. One that we tried was the Hugo Naturals Vanilla Sweet Orange shampoo which smelled great but didn't feel like it cleaned your hair. It didn't lather, as was the case with a few others we tried. But, as I mentioned, he and the kids have used shampoo bars ever since. There was only one thing remaining in his toilette that was of concern that I had overlooked (or, rather, had a hard time replacing) — his hairstyling product.

Hank had been using the same hairstyling product for years, American Crew Fiber. I gasped when I saw the ingredient list and immediately went on a search for an alternative. This product ranks a 9 out of a toxic 10 on the Environmental Working Group's Cosmetic Database for nasty ingredients like parabens, phthalates and, frankly, all sorts of crap. I could in no way let him put that anywhere near his skin again. Again, I turned to John Masters and was relieved to find they made a hair pomade that was similar to the one he was using. Again, it didn't work as well as the American Crew product and he complained that it looked like chicken grease, but it sure wasn't going to kill him.

I was still having difficulties finding any kind of styling product that was useful for me. Generally, I had been using hair-smoothing and straightening styling products that helped reduce frizz. Most of the natural products on the market were pretty simple and straightforward and didn't provide anything fancy like most conventional products. So I was happy to see that Whole Foods had started carrying some of the John Masters styling products besides just the hair pomade that my husband had been using. Some of the other styling products I had tried in the past that were organic or "natural" were awful.

At the risk of sounding like a shill for this product line, I found that the John Masters Sweet Orange & Silk Protein styling gel protected my hair from the hairdryer, did a decent enough job of keeping its hold and made my hair shiny and soft. More importantly, it smelled great and I knew it wasn't because it had a bunch of artificial fragrances in it. The underlying problem with finding hairstyling products is that there just aren't many natural nontoxic products on the market or, at least, they're not readily accessible. I think most manufacturers are focusing on the shampoo and conditioners and few have tackled the styling end of things. Or it could also possibly be that those individuals interested in "green" haircare products aren't as interested in styling products. In other words, there just isn't as much of a demand for them yet.

In the land of the moldy

Living in Seattle means there is a constant battle between good and evil. And by evil, I mean mold. And mildew and, just for kicks, you can toss in mushrooms as well. In every modern home that I've lived in here in the Pacific Northwest, we've always had issues with moisture. The combination of relative humidity and lack of sunlight means that nothing dries out for nine months of the year. There have been only two places that I lived that didn't have issues with mold and they were homes built over 100 years ago. In other words, they were drafty. They didn't have that airtight, energy-saving, heat-keeping tight frame you see in buildings built in the last 50 years or so. The end result is the newer the building, the worse the mold.

When I was growing up in the 1970s, our house (built around 1968 or so) was not just damp, it was cold. I remember always freezing in that house and it wasn't because my parents were doing some sort of blog challenge, they just kept the heat down. Couple that with the fact that the house was situated on top of some natural spring or stream or something and the end result was a lot of moisture inside. My childhood home is a bad example regarding moisture because we had, for a good portion of the year, a river of water literally running through the unfinished portion of our basement. You could open those wood louvered doors at the end of the family room and step into Ferngully down there with its strategically placed bricks, boards and other contraptions to get you from one end to the other without getting your feet too wet. Kind of like stepping stones through a stream but the hills were made out of black plastic tarp.

It was always my dad's fantasy to finish that end of the basement and he'd spin images of a giant playroom with a pool table and other such things. I'm pretty sure a wet bar was mentioned once or twice. Something the resident mice and other critters could really get into. The closest he got to any kind of drainage was building a sump pump in the front yard that never really took the edge off the flow. Any time there was a heavy rain, the laundry room got a deluge of water pouring through it. The basement smelled like a mix of must and mold which did wonders for my older brothers' asthma and allergies.

These two brothers, who still haven't let me live down the fact that I got the biggest (and, surely, the driest) bedroom in the house, were relegated to living in two of the three bedrooms that were in the "daylight" basement. We moved into this house right before I was born so I don't exactly recall all that went into their banishment to the basement, but suffice it to say that my dad did go so far as to finish two bedrooms and sort of a bathroom. Being more or less underground just meant that their bedrooms weren't exactly in the Sahara. And, because of the high moisture content down there, my brother Darryl routinely had interesting flora — of the fern kind — growing in his carpet.

That wasn't the last time I bore witness to things growing in the carpeting around here. When my husband and I were going to the University of Washington, we lived in an exceedingly cheap apartment in the University District in Seattle. This apartment was partially underground, so that when you looked out our bedroom window, you had to look up in order to see out. We didn't have much in the way of furniture in our living room, just a futon and an old heavy desk that Hank's father had managed to fashion out of what must be the heaviest wood found on planet Earth, or rather a mix of lead with a little plutonium. But the most offending object in that room was a television that we never watched and that was stuffed in the corner over by the sliding glass door that opened onto a one-foot-wide balcony.

Since these apartments were built on a slope, on one side we were underground and on the other we overlooked the street. Our balcony also overlooked the extremely noisy Knarr Tavern, which never had the door closed no matter the weather. The combination of jukebox and drunken pool table noise meant that we never had our sliding glass door open. This also meant that the air flow in that apartment was abysmal. We couldn't really afford to keep this place heated and visitors (of which we had few) complained that we could hang meat in there. Even though we didn't have too much of a mold problem, when we moved out after we graduated we noticed that we had created a bit of a terrarium in there by the glass door. As my husband went to move the television, he found a bumper crop of mushrooms growing under it.

I point this out only to show that Seattle, under the right conditions, can breed all sorts of internal plant and spore life if left unchecked. We didn't have anything spectacular going on in our current house even after the basement flooded a few years ago. A few hours with a wet/dry vacuum and some industrial fans for a few days cleared us of any problems. But we did have the classic windowsill mold in this house, just because they seal up tightly. Our last house had old, double-hung wood windows and we never had an issue with mold. Here, however, it was a constant battle. The other constant battle against mold was in our master bathroom. There's a window, but no fan.

The way the shower was constructed, it locked the moisture in the bathroom fairly well and did a slow release throughout the day. Our options were to leave the window open all day (which wasn't too pleasant in the winter) or get a fan installed. I'm sure you can guess by now that we haven't gotten around to getting a fan installed. It always got caught up in the whole, "let's remodel the bathroom if we are going to do that," which meant replacing the tiles, fixing the shower drip, installing the fan, replacing the vanity and getting new cabinets. The project always spun out of control and nothing ever got done, particularly since my husband got sick. And the last thing we wanted to endure was a bathroom remodel.

So, in order to assist the open window, I got a dehumidifier for the bathroom. It helped out immeasurably and I didn't need to deploy evasive mold tactics as often as I used to. But we still had mold both in the shower itself and on the walls. The only thing that worked on the tiles was bleach or some derivative product, like the heinous X-14. I'm fairly certain that I've shaved several years of lung and eye health off my life by using that stuff. You really do feel poisoned when you use it, but by gum, it works like a charm. As do most toxic products. I've tried a bevy of more natural solutions on the tiles including various mixtures containing one or more of the following: vinegar, hydrogen peroxide, borax, baking soda and tea tree oil, ad nauseum, but they all, frankly, don't do a damn thing. I've scrubbed and scrubbed and it's all for naught.

A few years ago I was sent a review sample of a product that cleans mold and mildew and is natural enough that the sales people are crazy enough to drink it just to show you how inert it truly is. The product, Concrobium Mold Control, is an off-the-shelf product that contains mostly inorganic compounds and leaves behind an antimicrobial film. This film, once dry, supposedly encapsulates fungus microbes and prevents their growth. This stuff works fairly well on the walls and lasts longer than the other options, but mold is mold and it always comes back.

I've tried Concrobium on the tiles and it doesn't really do much so we've been stuck using bleach. Going into this I knew, hands down, that this was going to be the hardest thing to find a natural replacement for. Because my husband and I both have back problems (his worse than mine due to the fact that his cancer has weakened and deteriorated his spine), putting in a little elbow grease to remove the mold or keep it in check isn't feasible. Bending over the shower to clean it will always result in a week spent flat-out with a bad back. So, our options are fairly limited.

I thought this would be one of those things in the project that we ended up failing on. Sticking with a light bleach spray is better than the alternative since the health risk of mold exposure isn't particularly good either. In this case it was a toss-up, unless I could find something off-the-shelf that wasn't toxic and actually worked. I went back to the Concrobium website to see if they had any hints on working with tiles. The walls weren't the issue and I felt like I had that part under control more or less. After rereading some tips, I gave the Concrobium another shot on the tiles and was consistent about using it.

The first thing we ended up doing to keep the mold on the tiles down was to keep the bathroom window open as long as feasible during the day. This did two things: it aired out the steam and kept the temperature of the bathroom relatively cool. Mold prefers a warm, moist environment. According to the product website, 70°–90°F is the sweet spot for mold growth. The second thing we did was to make sure the dehumidifier was running. This kept any remaining moisture from hanging around. Finally, I sprayed the Concrobium on the tiles once a week to prevent mold growth. Before I started this regimen I made sure the tiles got a good scrubbing and reduced the amount of mold as much as possible. It helped, but I still felt, after months, that we were swimming in mold overgrowth and resorted to a dilute bleach spray to knock it back again.

As far as the health effects of mold go, I'm not sure how it compares, overall, to the health effects of using bleach. Since my husband is immune-compromised not just because he is post-transplant but also because he takes immune suppressants *and* he's on a long-term chemotherapy drug, he is more susceptible to the health effects of mold which can cause infections and other respiratory problems. While we didn't have the toxic black mold (at least, I hope we didn't), any mold is not a good thing. It's about striking a balance between the risks of the problem and risks of the solution. One last thing—as soon as we added the tropical plants in the master bedroom and the bathroom, I noticed that the mildew smells decreased immensely. So much so that I went out and added an additional plant or two to that area.

Exercising with toxins

About a week before Thanksgiving, I was walking home from dropping the kids off at school and noticed that my left foot was bothering me. I had an injury in my left foot that had been off and on again for about a year. I had finally gone to see a podiatrist the previous spring and was diagnosed with sesamoiditis, which is the inflammation of a tiny bone the shape of a grain of rice in the ball of your foot. I was told to stay off it for a while and, in the meantime, the podiatrist added some cushioning to the insole of my walking shoes. It was a temporary fix that would last for a few weeks. He told me to come back and get some real orthotics made if that helped.

It did help and so I promptly ignored his suggestion of coming back, mostly because we were out of town for three weeks after my visit and the rest of the summer I was doing more yard work and less walking or running. When the school year started up I figured I should probably start exercising more. I had stopped exercising over that last year mostly because of the foot issue. In the spring I had taken up hula hooping, which was a great workout and didn't bother my foot, but I hadn't really been doing that either. So, I started walking every day after dropping the kids off at school. I tried to walk for at least 20 minutes, but I usually managed to go for 30 minutes before coming back home and writing.

During my morning walks, the conditions Dr. Hibbs and his staff had warned me about ran through my mind, mostly when a particularly odorous car drove by. Their warnings had to do with avoiding air pollution. I made sure I didn't walk out on the main roads, sticking to the residential streets that looped through my neighborhood. We don't get a lot of car traffic in our neighborhood, so my immediate exposure to toxic pollutants from car exhaust was less, but cars did drive by and I occasionally walked by someone smoking. Since it was fall, more people were burning wood so I could smell that too. And, although I love the smell of it, I had to wonder what I was breathing in.

During those months of walking, I let down my guard and wore some other shoes that tended to aggravate my foot problem. That, coupled with continued walking, just meant my sesamoid bone was getting more inflamed. I needed to find something else to do, at least to rest it in between walking and until I got some orthotics made. I decided on that trip home from school that I should dust off my hula hoop. The weather that day was extremely rainy and, although it wasn't currently raining, I figured hooping in the basement was better than doing it outside. Hooping with a lot of clothes on is virtually impossible, but hooping in our basement, with its low ceilings wasn't the best option either. It just meant that I had to stick to hooping on my body and not doing any fancy above-the-head tricks, which I like to do to work out my arms.

Unfortunately, while I was walking home I also remembered that I had made my hula hoop (as many people do) out of plastic tubing. I thought for sure that I had used PVC tubing, which meant that all that spare tubing I had stored in the laundry room was off-gassing polyvinyl chloride. And then there was the issue of the vinyl tape I used to wrap it and make it "sticky" for better grip. I figured if my hoop was toxic, I'd have to forgo using that as well and come up with something else to do for exercise. I could have ridden my bike, exposing myself to more pollutants from the car traffic, but the weather was just too windy and rainy and totally unmotivating. Biking would serve my purposes on days when there wasn't wind and driving rain and I could keep my biking limited to my neighborhood. It would just mean that I would be cycling around in circles a bit, but I figured that the once or twice a week bike ride when the weather cooperated would be fine.

I thought of swimming, but then I remembered about how the public pool I used is treated with chlorine and I would be exposed to all that off-gassing. The issue with chlorine-treated pools is that they off-gas chlorine and trichloramine, plus I'm sure you are absorbing some chlorine through your skin as well. Apparently, when the chlorine in pools reacts with organic materials like sweat and urine it can produce trichloramine (a lung irritant), which is then released into the air. These are really only a significant issue if the pool uses too much chlorine or if the smell of chlorine is strong in the air as it means there are high concentrations of trichloramines. The other option would be to use one of the local pools in the area that don't treat their pool water with chlorine, but they are all private pools and I didn't think it was necessarily worth the cost for a once a week swim.

When I got home, I looked up the type of tubing I had used in my hula hoop. For some reason I thought it was PVC, but PVC is too hard a plastic to use for a hula hoop. I had actually purchased and used polyethylene tubing instead. This is the type of tubing that is used for irrigation and is considered to be relatively non-toxic. High-density polyethylene(HDPE) is chlorine-free. PVC, on the other hand, contains chlorine, and dioxins are produced during the manufacture.[18] As far as I could tell, the tubing was fine. But what about the vinyl tape I used to wrap the tubing? That's where the problem was.

The 3M/Scotch Professional Grade electrical tape I used on it was made out of vinyl with a PVC backing. And not only was it vinyl but, being electrical tape, it was also a flame-retardant tape. If I stripped off the tape and replaced it with cloth tape, otherwise known as gaffers tape, then it would be good to go. But, since I had cross-wrapped the hoop with cloth tape that didn't come off too easily, I was better off making a new hoop out of the leftover HDPE tubing, wrapping it with cloth tape and then hanging my old hoop back up in the garage until I figured out what I wanted to do with it. Simple, right? Well, not so much. As I went to order cloth tape, it being relatively difficult to find in stores, I ran across this bit of information from hooptape.com. "Gaffers tape is made in lots of vibrant colors and it has a vinyl coating, which makes it colorfast and easy to wipe clean."

After doing a bit of digging online, mostly on websites catering to people who have latex allergies, someone suggested using colored athletic tape. What I did find was a paucity of information about the tapes and, after finding some cloth hockey-stick tape that looked like it fit the bill and didn't announce that it was vinyl impregnated like the cloth gaffers tape, I ended up emailing the company to be sure. They wrote back and said that the tape was, indeed, free of vinyl. It was a cotton and polyester blend, so I could continue hooping with a non-toxic hoop. I just needed to make a new one.

Other indoor options were watching exercise DVDs or using our treadmill. I found neither of these very enthralling and that is why I was walking outside. I couldn't use the treadmill for obvious foot issues, but I could see what Netflix had in the way of workout DVDs. I hadn't explored the toxins in electronics as yet. In a perfect world, I'd be walking and biking outside (on clean air days) and swimming in a nonchlorine pool for my exercise. I really didn't figure that staying in shape would expose me to so many potential additional toxins. After all that, it made me want to just stay on the couch.

Moles in my molehill

Speaking of couch, I can't help but be reminded that our front lawn, for a few weeks in November, had been slowly turning into molehill central. It started one weekend with two dirt lumps popping up near the fig tree. When I went for a walk that day I was at least pleased to see that we weren't the only ones sporting dirty lumps in our lawn. The neighbors on either side of us were each afflicted with their own pair of molehills. Over the next few days, I would wake up to another molehill and then another. It got to the point that every morning we were greeted by an additional molehill, all in a linear path heading out to the street. By the time a week had passed, we had eight dirt piles in our lawn and it was time to take some action.

I looked into what could be causing the hilling. I didn't think we had many burrowing animals in our area and narrowed it down to the rather populous (at least in Seattle and the Pacific Northwest) Townsend's mole, aka *Scapanus townsendii*. The evidence left behind seemed to match the criminal profile. It could also have been a gopher, but they are relatively rare around Seattle. A Townsend's mole, which is 8–9 inches long and black in color, has a general population density with the typical city lot containing one or two moles.[19] Why we've never had them before is surprising although I've seen plenty of neighbors' lawns exhibiting signs of inhabitants.

According to Sunrise Pest Management, Townsend's moles feed primarily on insect larvae, earthworms, slugs, centipedes, roots and seeds. We certainly had an abundance of those things in our front lawn. When I was searching for solutions to our mole issues, I ran across a laundry list of things that people do to try to deter them, ranging from using poison, insecticides and smoke bombs to burying razor blades. I didn't want to kill or trap the mole and I certainly didn't want to poison the little fella, even if he was making a mess of my yard. Any chemical agent or poison surely would affect not only wildlife but also the environment, as the runoff from our yard goes directly out to Puget Sound and I couldn't imagine what mole bait and kill would do to the local fish populations.

Sunrise Pest Management does do an environmentally (and critter-friendly) treatment using a natural treatment that makes

---

Homemade Mole Control

The formula for the castor-oil repellent can be made by using a blender to combine ¼ cup of unrefined castor oil (can be purchased at most pharmacies) and 2 tablespoons of a dishwashing liquid. Blend the two together, add 6 tablespoons water, and blend again. Combine the concentrated mixture with water at a rate of 2 tablespoons of solution to 1 gallon of water. Use a watering can or sprayer to liberally apply the solution to areas where moles are active. The above mixture will cover approximately 300 square feet.

The repellent will be most effective where it can be watered into the moist soil surrounding surface tunnels made by moles. Areas that receive extensive irrigation will quickly lose the repellent to leaching. For best results, spray the entire area needing protection; moles will burrow under a perimeter treatment.

The repellent may need to be reapplied before moles depart. Once moles move elsewhere, the solution usually remains effective for 30 to 60 days.

Courtesy of WDFW (wdfw.wa.gov/living/moles.html)

---

the mole's food source taste bitter. Since the moles don't like Sour Patch worms, they leave in search of other food. Better still, the worms and other insects are unharmed. I sent Sunrise an email to get a quote and see if it was worth the cost to have them come out and do an initial treatment. If it was going to be expensive, I figured I'd just rake over the mounds, stamp down the tunnels and hope for the best. It's not like our pesticide-free lawn was immaculate in the first place. Since we've never used synthetic chemicals, herbicides or pesticides on our yard, the lawn was already pretty lumpy.

Another option was a homemade castor oil–based treatment that I found on the Washington State Department of Fish & Wildlife website. They claimed the treatment rendered the mole's prey distasteful and, if eaten, would give the moles diarrhea. I guess it's better than instant death. When I got the response from Sunrise, I found out that they used a castor oil–based treatment as well so I decided that if the problem continued I was going to save myself the money and go with this completely non-toxic, cheap, homemade treatment instead.

Going BPA bananas

In mid-November, I received an email from my editor at New Society Publishers with a link to a study on how BPA is absorbed by the skin. I had been seeing this mentioned increasingly over the previous several weeks, mostly in relation to store receipts. As soon as I read the reports I had become a little bit crazy about handling store receipts and almost dreaded it when the cashier handed one to me. I never exactly planned ahead about what to do with it and I ended up treating it like a hot potato, dropping it into my reusable bag filled with my purchases or, worse, putting it into my purse where it would be touched again and again until I removed it and put it somewhere else. I ended up just making sure that I was wearing my gloves by the time they handed it to me and, if it wasn't cold enough to wear gloves, I made sure I washed my hands as soon as I could.

Bisphenol-A, the latest bad boy chemical in the news, is known as an estrogen mimic. According to French scientists, it can readily pass through the skin by way of cash register receipts. Three studies showed that BPA is found in a large percentage of receipts in the U.S. and can rub off onto your hands. In a separate survey of 400 pregnant women, it was found that the highest BPA concentrations were found in cashiers.[20]

Now, I'm in no way a cashier, and I don't spend much time buying things, but if I'm going to go out of my way to avoid touching, ingesting or inhaling various toxins, then I sure don't like being duped into BPA exposure when I go shopping. While Canada has recognized BPA as being toxic, the U.S. hasn't done much in the way of regulating it. Several states have made efforts to limit the chemical in baby and kids' products, but it's still very much available as a lining in cans as well as in other hard plastics. Until better regulation of the substance occurs, I'll be the crazy lady in line at the grocery store handling her receipt with a pair of salad tongs.

Heating with PFCs

Right before Thanksgiving, I ran across a post on the Safer Chemicals, Healthy Families Facebook page. The person who posted the message had mentioned how she was considering purchasing a microwave that also served as an oven but was concerned because it was lined with Teflon. I hadn't even thought about the possible nonstick surfaces in our microwave. I looked at the interior and it certainly had a hard plastic look to it, but I wasn't sure if it was made with PFCs so I decided to do a little digging.

At first I thought, if it were a problem, I would just reheat things on the stovetop. It's less convenient and not as energy efficient if I have to reheat things in the oven rather than the microwave, but I was willing to do it. And then I looked at my cook top and figured it also had some sort of nonstick surface on it. Then I thought the same thing about the interior of the oven. Ack! I couldn't exactly cook on a wood stove or propane grill or anything—the toxins from those probably weren't that much better. It was time to do some more research.

We were in the process of finally installing an over-the-oven microwave that we had purchased, ahem, five years before. That particular microwave had a stainless steel interior. But it still wasn't installed. What about the stand-alone one we had been using? As I mentioned, it looked to have some plastic-type interior, but I couldn't find any information about it. As for our GE convection range, the cook top (one of those smooth-top radiant surface units) was actually made out of some sort of "black glass ceramic." As for the interior, I really couldn't find any information about what it was made out of. I suspect it was also some sort of porcelain coating, but I really didn't know.

So, in all honesty—I gave up trying to find out. I didn't exactly have any feasible alternatives anyway and my research was going nowhere fast. I decided to assume that all was right with our cooking apparati that none of them had any kind of Teflon- or PFC-impregnated surfaces or linings. I couldn't find anything to suggest that any of them did, which was a good thing since heating up those surfaces to the temperatures we normally do would have created a whole lot of off-gassing.

Dishwasher

While I was focused on the kitchen, I was reminded about the dishwasher. Around Halloween, our relatively new dishwasher, which was installed right before we moved in five years before, decided to sound like it was on its last legs. Occasionally, when we ran a load, it made the most horrific noise for the duration of the cycle. On top of that, the top rack decided to pop a wheel and lose a few other useful parts. We ordered a new one with a stainless steel exterior and interior to minimize the heating up of plastic pieces. As a result, I had little to worry about as far nonstick lining in the dishwasher went. But the dishwasher detergent was something to reinvestigate.

A year before we got our new dishwasher, we had made the

switch from commercial dishwashing detergent to something more environmentally friendly for several reasons. The first was the impact of phosphate-laden dishwashing detergent on wildlife. The problem with phosphates is that they act like a fertilizer, increasing algae and weed growth in waterways. Wastewater treatment plants can't remove the phosphorous from detergents that end up in the sewage. When treated wastewater (still containing the phosphates) is discharged out into Puget Sound or other waterways, the resulting algal and weed growth can deplete the oxygen needed by fish and other aquatic life downstream. Since we made the switch, Washington State had enacted a ban on phosphates in dishwashing detergent.

The second issue with our previous detergent was the amount of plastic it used. The products we were using were the liquid detergents in the big plastic bottles and it always seemed like we were going through a lot of detergent, and therefore bottles, since we ran the dishwasher every day. Even recycling the plastic containers didn't make the impact seem less of an issue and, if we were going to try to find a powdered detergent in a cardboard box, I figured we might as well try to find one without phosphates as well as one that had minimal impact on the environment.

Trying to find a dishwashing detergent with low or no phosphates isn't very difficult. The hard part is trying to find one that actually works. Phosphates are what make the surfactants in the detergent work well. We went through several different brands before finally stumbling upon one that we liked, Ecover Dishwasher Tablets. The tablets came in a cardboard box and the only plastic used was in a thin film covering the individual tablets, and at least it was recyclable. More importantly, the tablets actually worked just as well as the commercial products we were using before. Products like Electrasol and Cascade.

One thing that was noticeable when we started using the Ecover tablets was that, when we ran the dishwasher, it didn't smell. That overpoweringly strong smell that used to emanate from the dishwasher and that smelled like hot cleaner and bleach was no longer there. Now there was no smell at all. And I felt like I could breathe in the kitchen with the dishwasher running.

The biggest danger in using commercial dishwashing detergent is that most of them generally contain dry chlorine. When dissolved in water, the dry chlorine is activated and those chlorine fumes in the steam that smells-up the kitchen can cause eye irritation and breathing difficulties. Chlorine bleach can also combine with carbon molecules which, in turn, can create organochlorines such as dioxin, a known carcinogen. Additionally, detergents may contain artificial fragrance (phthalates) as well as quarternium 15, which is an irritant and allergen that can also release the carcinogenic formaldehyde.[21] All this gives new meaning to the word and product "Cascade." Breathing in all that airborne junk was not really my idea of fresh and clean, so I was quite happy to have circumvented the problem altogether.

Clean eating

Once this project was underway and I had had my initial body burden testing done, I slowly started introducing more organic foods into my diet. Even before, I normally ate a lot of organic foods, but over the months following the tests, I really went out of my way to make sure that the food I was eating was organic. I was trying to avoid pesticides like the plague and eating organic was one of the quickest ways to guarantee their avoidance. This meant that every shopping trip became one of analysis for the first several weeks. It was difficult to break out of the pattern and rhythm of just grabbing the same products that I was used to. For the most part, it really wasn't all that difficult to replace items with an organic version of the same thing. The difficult part was when I craved something *in particular* that wasn't organic.

The last problem I dealt with in regards to food consumption had to do with avoiding BPA in cans. I really didn't eat too many canned items to begin with, but there were a couple staples I needed to remind myself to avoid—canned refried beans and black olives. Finding organic canned refried beans isn't a problem, but

finding them in a non-BPA can was difficult. There's one manufacturer, Eden Organics, that sells refried beans in a BPA-free can
but I'd have to order a case online and we just don't eat enough of it
to warrant the purchase. Organic canned olives are nearly impossible to find in our regular grocery store, so I would have to go to a
specialty store. Most likely the can would have a BPA plastic lining
anyway. So, I just decided to forgo black olives and use dried beans
instead of refried, which wasn't exactly a big deal. I also wasn't
eating tuna because of the mercury and arsenic, so that wasn't an
issue either. The only thing I stopped altogether that I had been
eating occasionally was canned organic soup. Again, it was just
something to pay attention to but I wasn't exactly depriving myself.

The hardest thing about changing my diet had more to do with
eating out or going to coffee shops. I can't say that, for the first two
months of the project, we went out to eat much. We went out a
few times here and there, but I wasn't focusing as much on the
food so I let it slide. As the months passed, I started to really think
about it, and it made going out to eat much more of an impossibil-
ity. There are only a few restaurants with organic or sustainably
grown food on the menus and generally those aren't the places the
kids want to go. In other words, they are more along the lines of
fine dining establishments.

Going out to coffee shops was much more difficult to avoid
because it's something we do a lot of. Several of the ones in our
area offer organic milk and some organic baked goods and many
of the places we go to serve organic, fair trade coffee. But few offer
all three and we went to those places maybe half the time. I think
I was starting to annoy my husband, who is Mr. Coffee Shop
Extraordinaire, with my limitations. He was getting sick of my
few selections. Even if the place sold organic coffee, they generally
didn't offer organic milk. Not having food there wasn't a problem,
I didn't mind just going for the coffee. So I just started drinking
Americanos (which is just espresso and hot water) because then
I could skip the milk if they didn't have an organic option. And,
when it came down to it, most places had organic tea, which I

would choose instead. The only problem is that it meant I didn't actually get to eat anything. Which just meant that I sometimes came home hungry from our outings.

Winter gardening

As the weather started getting colder and crappier, my husband asked me if it was possible to still grow some vegetables in the garden over the winter. We had gotten spoiled with our vegetable CSA, which was about to end, and with going out in our backyard to grab vegetables and herbs whenever we felt like it. The funny thing was, I had just been thinking about how to create some sort of greenhouse over our raised beds without too much trouble. This would extend our growing season to year round with access to almost 30 different kinds of vegetables that don't require heat or much in the way of daylight, particularly in our area where it is dark but not incredibly cold. Well, not Maine cold, even if we were supposed to have a colder winter than usual. Temperatures below freezing are relatively rare, even this far north since we live in a fairly temperate area.

Since I was already spending some time out back this year with our chickens in the way of feeding, watering and collecting eggs, it wouldn't take much more effort to tend to a winter garden. Even without any kind of protection over the crop, by late November I was still collecting enough salad greens for a few large salads per week. The rest of the vegetables were more or less at the end of their lives, but the radishes and the beets were still plugging along. With more of a greenhouse environment, the interior temperatures would be higher and the yield would go up. Plus, I could continue planting throughout the rest of the fall and into the winter.

After doing a bit of research, I decided that installing mini hoop houses over the beds seemed to be the way to go. Initially I was seeing that a lot of people used metal tubing that they bent over the beds and then covered in some sort of greenhouse plastic (similar to a covered wagon). The metal seemed like a huge pain in the behind but people used it because it held up to heavy snowfall.

Since we rarely get snow, it seemed like a bit of overkill, so when I read that others just use PVC or HDPE flexible irrigation tubing, I just about jumped for joy because I had a lot of irrigation tubing still hanging out in my basement, waiting to be made into hula hoops.

Since I had already done some reconnaissance on the irrigation tubing in reference to my hula hoop toxicity, I knew that the hoop parts of the mini hoop houses were safe. I wasn't about to use the PVC. But, what about the greenhouse plastic sheeting people were recommending? That sounded to me like vinyl. As it turned out, it is commonly made from polyethylene (HDPE) just like my irrigation tubing. I was also concerned that the impermeable covering would mean I would need to actually either water the beds or set up some sort of irrigation instead of taking advantage of the free rainfall we were getting. Because of that I looked into getting some HDPE fabric covering that allows the rain to come in, but helps keep out heavy rain and wind. All I needed was some clips and we were good to go for an extended season of organic, pesticide-free gardening.

Watch out

I hated my new watch. I had replaced my old watch at the beginning of this project because I figured it wasn't exactly the most non-toxic thing that I wear every day, for hours a day. The watch that I used to wear had a stainless steel backing, but the rest of it was a combination of hard, soft and molded plastic. The watchband was also made out of a bendable, vinyl plastic, similar to a rubber duck, which I was afraid was chock-full of phthalates. In addition to the plastic casing, body and band on my watch, the battery inside was a standard mercury battery. Mercury is a neurotoxin and exposure to even small amounts of mercury over a long period may cause negative health effects including damage to the brain, kidney and lungs, and to a developing baby. I didn't need to worry about that last part, but I wanted to keep damage to my organs at a minimum.

I managed to find a watch that avoided these problems. It was made by Sprout, and, like all the other watches they manufacture, it was in compliance with the *Consumer Product Safety Improvement Act* (CPSIA) and was lead- and phthalate-free. The watch face was made from bamboo and the watch casing itself was made from corn resin. The watch band was woven from organic cotton and the lens was constructed of mineral crystal, rather than plastic. Finally, Sprout uses only mercury-free batteries.

When I ordered it online from Amazon, I was delighted that the watch wasn't hideous and had some extra neat features that my old sports watch didn't have. Plus, it was still water resistant, so I didn't feel like I was giving up any features from my previous watch. In fact, I felt I was gaining something in having not only a non-toxic watch, but a very environmentally friendly one as well, which was most likely going to be a conversation piece, too. Boy, was I wrong.

First of all, I loved the fact that it was all non-toxic and environmentally friendly, as I suspected I would. But I hated the fact that the thing was huge. Honking big huge. From the looks of it online and the description of it being a women's watch, complete with purple watch band and a cute little birdie on the watch face, you'd think it would be dainty. But it was the size of a man's watch. A manly man's watch—which was okay once I got used to the size. Everything else appeared as advertised with the corn resin watch with the cotton strap and the bamboo parts of the face. All lead-, phthalate- and mercury-free. What could go wrong?

Well, the watch face had some problems. Maybe it was my eyes. No, it wasn't my eyes, because my husband had the same problem. I couldn't see anything on the watch face. All the mini dials were too small to see, even with my glasses on. With my glasses off, there was no chance at all. That meant that the 24-hour dial, the day of the week and the day of the month dials were impossible to see unless I held it real close to my face and squinted and as long as the lighting was good. Because of the way the hands were built, you couldn't see them against the background, because the background was too shiny.

In any case, all this meant was that most of the time I was wearing it I had no idea what the actual time was and absolutely no idea what the date was. And it drove me bonkers. But I didn't want to go back to a watch that had a plastic case or a mercury battery, which would include all my other watches, including my stainless steel one.

Going
a Little Bonkers

Leaving the sanctuary

I didn't get out much during those first few months of the project. Since I was working from home, I didn't have to deal with foreign hand soap at work or exposure to perfumes and fragrances from co-workers. I basically dropped the kids off at school and picked them up again. My interactions with people were mostly outside and my exposure to any products was minimal. Sometimes I'd be overwhelmed by someone's perfume in the school during pickup and I couldn't help thinking that I was inhaling a wall of phthalates. I even went so far as to hold my breath, although I doubt that did anything besides make me look more weird than usual.

Going out to stores posed the same problem. I was exposed to more perfumes, products and overly scented this and that. These are things that I'm normally sensitive to and now I was beyond annoyed by their presence. I suppose I could have limited myself to stores such as Whole Food or our local co-op, PCC, as the exposure would be less, but sometimes I needed to buy something else or didn't want to pay the Whole Foods prices for the same products at our other stores.

I knew I had a problem when one day we were all out at the store picking up a few items and I realized I needed to go to the bathroom. It couldn't wait until we got home since we were also stopping by the store next door on the way back. We were at our local Fred Meyer store in Seattle, a store we refer to as "Dirty Fred's" just because it's one of the grubbier Fred Meyer stores in town and there's a nasty-smelling hotdog cart in the entrance. The bathrooms are kind of skanky in spite of being newly spruced up, and I hate going in there because of the hand soap they use. This is the case at all the Fred Meyer stores in Seattle; they must all use the same industrial soap. This stuff stinks and, worse yet, it lingers for hours afterwards.

The thought of the hand soap crossed my mind and I actually deliberated not going to the bathroom just to avoid The Soap. Knowing that I probably wouldn't make it, though, I decided to use the bathroom, but not the soap. I would scrub my hands thoroughly with warm water. Since I knew we were going home soon, I figured it wouldn't make that much difference. I know plenty of people who, as a rule, don't wash their hands after going to the bathroom. At least I had a legitimate reason — I didn't want to have some potentially triclosan-, paraben- and phthalate-laden soap on my hands.

At that point, I realized this was going to be a problem whenever we went out to stores, and especially restaurants. So I bought a little travel-size bottle of liquid soap (actually a shower gel) from one of my favorite manufacturers. It was the Hugo Naturals Vanilla Sweet Orange gel. I figured I could get away with carrying it around and if anyone asked why I was using my own soap I figured that, instead of explaining the whole ordeal, I would just claim an allergy. It would save time and it wouldn't be the first time I'd used that excuse in the course of trying to get more information for this project. But then I started thinking that maybe it would be useful as an educational moment. If someone asked me, I could explain why. But it's so convoluted and, with most people completely unaware of the crap they slather on themselves every day, I would most certainly come off sounding like a kook. I would need to work on my chemical message.

One evening I went to a cast member and crew get-together to talk more about the makeover show I was a cast member on,

Mission: Sustainable, and how we were going to continue working on the show by making webisodes to keep people interested in the environmental message we had introduced with the pilot episode. My role on the show is Personal Care Consultant and I do make-overs on items from personal care products to cleaning supplies and soaps to paper products and everything in between.

Not knowing what kind of food and drink was going to be there, I dutifully brought over a bottle of organically grown grape-based wine and planned to not eat anything. Fortunately, much of the food was from a local farmers' market and I could more or less assume that minimal pesticides were used. Even the cheese was safe. There was one dish, in spite of looking fantastic and having all the elements of tastiness about it — garlic, rosemary, olive oil — that I had to keep reminding myself to not eat. It was made from nonorganic canned beans and I couldn't help but look at it and think, "Bowl of BPA!" There were a few other things I also had to make a conscious effort to avoid, but all in all, it was a success.

A success until I went to wash my hands, that is. I had a few choices in the kitchen — a liquid soap pump dispenser and a Seventh Generation Dishwashing Liquid bottle. Since I didn't have my glasses on, it wasn't until after I pumped the liquid soap that I realized I should have gone with the giant dishwashing liquid bottle. I made sure the next time I washed my hands that, even if it looked weird that I was using the big bottle, I used the one that I knew was "safe."

The hostess, Becky, remarked midway through our get-together that her wife was concerned about having us over because we would be critical of some non-environmentally friendly things they had in the house. It makes sense. I mean, we were hired for the show to go into people's homes to do a makeover — to find things they were using or doing that weren't sustainable or environmentally friendly and challenge them to change their behaviors. Our producer quickly replied, "We wouldn't do that!" and

Becky blurted out, "Deanna!" I guess she was concerned I would go sniffing through their bathroom or something which, I have to admit, is hard for me not to do when I go over people's homes.

It's not that I'm that nosy, I'm just curious to see how environmentally "enlightened" people are or not. I don't expect someone from the general public to have made any changes, but I do have high expectations for people who focus on environmentalism. It goes with the territory. I spend so much of my time thinking about environmentally unfriendly habits and non-sustainable or dangerous products that it's hard for me not to have that carry over to everywhere I go and everything I do. It's a little annoying, but I generally never say anything unless someone asks me. And I don't bombard them with "you should's." I much prefer to gently educate by answering questions, pointing out things and explaining what the potential problems are. Offering alternatives and acknowledging that it's difficult to make changes goes a long way in getting the idea across. Much better than the sledgehammer approach.

Stuck in the sink

I was dreading the part of the project where I needed to really analyze our drain-cleaning situation. I hadn't yet found a decent alternative to unclogging drains, which is a huge problem in our house. I don't know if it's because we have plumbing issues, kids who put too much crap down the sink or too much hair, but it always seems like something is backed up. Over the years, I've tried a number of different solutions instead of our old standby Liquid-Plumr. I've tried the baking soda and vinegar option. I've tried the baking soda and vinegar, followed by boiling water option. I've tried the prophylactic use of both, but it really only slows down the inevitable arrival of Liquid-Plumr. It's a love-hate relationship — mostly hate.

I hate the fact that it's toxic, containing a combination of sodium hydroxide and sodium hypochlorite (that's lye and bleach). This doesn't sit well with me. So, I've also tried this contraption that looks like a long piece of plastic with hooks on the side that is supposed to grab and pull up whatever is clogging your drains. I bought it and used it and it grabbed absolutely nothing. I tried it on several different drains in hopes that it would unclog the giant hairball/Lego/paper wads that were lurking in the sink, but to no avail. I had such high hopes for it, but I was so frustrated and disappointed with this contraption that I threw it in the trash.

This time around, I tried a "natural enzyme" product that was supposed to do something similar to Draino or Liquid-Plumr—that is, eat away at the clog. The problem with the product I bought, Earth Friendly Products' Earth Enzymes, is that you have to mix the solution, pour it in and wait 24 hours. This is not a product for someone in a hurry or someone who needs to have access to the sink or drain you are trying to unclog. But, in the spirit of trying out all my options, I finally gave it a whirl. Or, rather, my husband kept bugging me to use it otherwise he was going to reach for the Draino.

We invested the 24 hours in our bathroom sink. I followed the directions to a T to make sure I gave it a fair shake. I mixed the solution, poured it in, waited 24 hours and even flushed it with boiling water at the end. Did it work? It didn't do a damn thing. The drain was just as clogged as it was 24 hours prior. The main ingredients in the Earth Enzymes are sodium sesquicarbonate, bacterial mixtures and proteolytic enzymes. Sodium sesquicarbonate is similar to baking soda so it doesn't surprise me that it didn't do much more than the baking soda/vinegar solution. Actually, I take that back—baking soda and vinegar worked better. And they were less expensive and time-consuming.

After all that I decided to just try straight-up lye since I had it in the house anyway. I would at least be reducing the bleach usage. What I wanted to know was, why did we stop using lye as a drain cleaner and start using the lye/bleach combo that is in Draino and Liquid-Plumr? Was it because it was more effective? Were these new products initially powder or liquid? In any case, drain cleaning has gotten more caustic and toxic over the years. To truly clean out one's pipes in a non-toxic way, getting a drain snake is in order, but

I gather that few people are willing to mess with that. We sure as hell aren't.

Lip locked

A few years ago I started having an incredibly strange allergic reaction to some lip balm or lipstick I was using. It took me a while to figure out what was going on, but by the time I stopped using it, my lips were more or less unhappy with me. They were slightly swollen and burning and tingling for about a month, at which point they decided to peel. And peel. And peel. I'm not the only one this has happened to, as some of my blog readers wrote in to commiserate with me. I never did find out what the offending ingredient was but I was sure to avoid the products that were causing me grief.

At the time the only thing that wasn't bothering my lips was straight-up petroleum jelly. I also managed to have success with a random trial of a Cover Girl cocoa-mint lip gloss that I really liked. Until I found out what it had in it (parabens and propylene glycol) and then I stopped using it over the summer. When I was rehabbing my makeup and falling in love with Gabriel Cosmetics, I figured I could get away with using one of his lip glosses. I found one that had the same color and look as the Cover Girl and figured I was set. I used it infrequently, but the one week that I decided to use it a couple times, I started having the same reaction again.

For days my lips felt numb with a burning and tingling sensation that was literally driving me crazy. One morning, in a bit of a stupor, I reached for some hydrocortisone cream. I congratulated myself for thinking of this because I had been suffering for a few days and figured that, if this were an allergic reaction to something in the lip gloss, then the cream would help. It wasn't until the second application that I decided I should probably look at the ingredient list. I had convinced myself that it just contained hydrocortisone and nothing else. I should have known better.

In addition to the active ingredient, there were a few other things that made me kick myself for trying it—methylparaben, propylparaben, propylene glycol, liquid paraffin and sodium cetearyl sulfate. I suppose a little parabens weren't going to kill me, but I felt this screw-up was far worse than some of the other things I accidentally used or ate or chose to continue using. I threw out the hydrocortisone cream and stuck with my favorite Badger Lip Balm.

However, I just so happened to be at the store researching new drain openers when I decided to see if they had a tinted Badger Lip Balm, since I'd seen it there in the past and figured I'd try it out. They, in fact, did sell it and I ended up bringing home a double-ended lip tint and shimmer that I was excited to try out. Big mistake. Whatever was in the Badger tinted balm was even worse than whatever was in the Gabriel gloss and my lips were even more tingly and irritated. I'm talking about a 24-hour-a-day sensation.

I went back through the ingredients of both products to see if I could finally figure out what the problem was. I was able to get an ingredient list on the Cover Girl Wetslicks product to cross-reference the ingredients and narrow down the offending ones, but I still couldn't figure out what the problem was. So it was back to plain Badger. I never did find out what the problem was with these two mostly natural products. It's funny that the one product (Cover Girl) that was chock-full of chemicals didn't cause a reaction, but the ones that were natural did.

Laminated turkeys

The week before Thanksgiving my daughter brought home a Thanksgiving-themed placemat that she had made at school. She was very proud of and excited about it and wanted to use it the second we got home for her snack. I didn't mind, but I couldn't help wondering the whole time what exactly the laminating film was made out of. I really didn't think it was made out of vinyl or PVC or anything like that but I certainly didn't want her food touching some potentially nasty plastic since she tends to take things out of bowls and eat directly off the placemat.

After doing some initial research on the laminating film and machines commonly used in schools and offices, I found out that the film was made out of either some sort of co-polymer or a polyester film. Based on how nonrigid the placemat was, I concluded it was made out of polyester with an adhesive layer of polyethelene. While I didn't really want her eating off something artificial or plastic (we had gotten rid of all our plastic kitchen dishes and cups months before), I figured she'd only use it for a week or less. Since it was polyester it wouldn't do much harm for the short term. There are some cold-laminating films made out of PVC, but given the fact that the placemat wasn't stiff I didn't think it was made from that. I had already started making her overly aware of chemicals and so I let this one slide lest I drive her completely crazy with worry.

Snow and toothpaste

The first day of Thanksgiving break we had a bit of a snowstorm. What that meant was that our schedules got jumbled around, our parent-teacher conferences were cancelled and the kids were clamoring to get outside and play in this relatively uncommon event for Seattle. All this distraction also meant that I wasn't paying attention when I put toothpaste on my toothbrush that morning. Instead of going for the Tom's of Maine SLS-free toothpaste that I had switched over to for the last two months, I accidentally grabbed my husband's Colgate toothpaste. I figured it wasn't that big a deal, they both had fluoride in them, with the only real difference being that Tom's lacks sodium lauryl sulfates (SLS), which makes the toothpaste foamy. My husband couldn't get over the lack of lather in the Tom's so he continued using the Colgate.

Sodium lauryl sulfate ranks a 3 out of 10 for toxicity on the Environmental Working Group's Cosmetic Database for being a potential toxin. As far as I can tell the jury is still out on this ingredient, but it's something I try to avoid in my personal care products, particularly with things that go in my mouth. As for the fluoride, I am still ambivalent about this ingredient in my toothpaste. And I'm not swallowing it, unlike our water. At least, I'm not intentionally swallowing it. I make sure I rinse thoroughly and keep the fluoride where it is potentially helping the most—on my teeth. Although the specific Tom's toothpaste I was using wasn't ranked on the cosmetic database, based on its ingredient list, I figured it was between a 2 and a 3 (because of the fluoride).

My husband, on the other hand, is in dire need of extra fluoride for a number of reasons. He even has additional tubes of fluoride in the cabinet that goes straight on, although I don't think he uses it as often as he needs to. One of the medications he used to take for his cancer can cause bone loss in the jaw and so it is imperative that his teeth get enough fluoride. Any dental work can be a catastrophe (causing jaw necrosis or death to the jaw bone), so keeping his teeth healthy is crucial. And that requires more fluoride than the average person needs. My only dental issue is a result of grinding while I sleep and no amount of fluoride is going to stop me from doing that.

In any case, I wondered how badly the plain old Colgate that I used that morning ranked since it wasn't the fancy product with extra whitening, tartar control and whatnot. It turned out it only ranked a 4 out of 10, mostly for the fluoride, SLS and artificial flavor. Since the Tom's of Maine uses a naturally sourced fluoride, similar to the kind used in Colgate, between the SLS-free business and lack of artificial flavorings, Tom's of Maine in general was ranked just a little bit lower. Even though the differential was small (it wasn't like it was an 8 versus a 2) and even though I prefer Colgate, I stuck with the Tom's without other artificial ingredients and SLS.

Now, when compared to the Aquafresh Bubble Mint that my kids like, the Tom's stood out more. Not only did the Aquafresh get a ranking of 5, mostly for the combo of SLS, fluoride and flavorings, it also had a 9 ranking for the type of fluoride used, which was a concern. And it contained some PEGs and a host of artificial colorings. My kids were pretty good about not swallowing toothpaste, but I can't say that I really trusted them not to eat it on occasion because they had done it in the past. Getting them to switch toothpaste was a bit of a problem, but I managed to get Henry to switch to a combo of Tom's and Colgate so, at the very least, his exposure to some of the artificial ingredients and nastier fluoride source was reduced. It took months but I eventually switched both Emma and Henry exclusively over to Tom's.

Missing labs

It had been almost two months since I had gotten my labs done and I still hadn't gotten back the results for the combined panel for perchlorinated pesticides, PCBs, DDTs and the like. At that point I was hoping they hadn't gotten lost because I had already drastically reduced the amount of pesticide exposure I was ingesting by eating an almost 100% organic diet. It was difficult to do, to say the least, especially on the occasions that we ate out, but I couldn't fathom losing those initial results to see if all the trouble was even worth it.

I followed up with Dr. Hibbs just to make sure that he hadn't accidentally overlooked any test results that may have come in and just forgotten to forward them to me. Unfortunately, that wasn't the case—he had never received the results. He sent an email to the lab to see if they had gotten anything from Metametrix. In the meantime, I continued my strict eating and hoped that I didn't have to go without those data points. The PCB and DDT levels in my body probably hadn't changed drastically up until then since they are stored in fat and I hadn't been doing too much yet to purge fat-soluble toxins from my system. However, I still wanted to know what the starting level was.

Cancer update

At the end of November, my husband was still on an ongoing treatment of Revlimid, the chemotherapy drug that is targeted to damage his cancer cells but keep his healthy cells, well, healthy. There is a relatively easy blood test that he has done once a month or so to check for cancer markers. The definitive method for testing his cancer levels is a series of bone marrow biopsies, but those are painful and pretty invasive (they essentially drill a few holes in my husband's pelvis and suck out the marrow). The blood test, which checks for this thing called an M-spike, gives you a pretty decent idea of what's going on in the bone marrow without having to crack it open.

My husband's cancer, multiple myeloma, is characterized by malignant plasma cells that reproduce uncontrollably. These plasma cells produce excessive monoclonal proteins, or M proteins. Checking for the M protein in your blood tells you how much malignancy (or cancer) you have coursing through your bone marrow and, therefore, through your blood. It's a pretty handy test to have and certainly can help you get a good idea of where you are, cancer-wise.

Back in September, when they tested Hank, his M-spike was at .4 g/dl (that's grams per deciliter). In October, it went down to .3 g/dl. During Hank's October visit with his oncologist, Dr. Benziger, they talked a little about my book and what we were doing around the house to lower our exposure to toxins. His doctor joked that the drop in his M-spike had something to do with my toxin removal program. I'm sure it had much more to do with his chemotherapy, but I was also sure that Hank's system not being bombarded by a bunch of toxins gave it the extra bandwidth to deal with the cancer cells. We'll never know, of course, what all was contributing to his numbers going lower, but we didn't care. They were lower and that's what mattered.

In Hank's November tests, his blood work looked good and they were able to reduce one of the immune suppressants he was on even further. Hank had been on these suppressants (drugs like Prednisone and Tacrolimus) post-stem cell transplant as it is very common for the new immune system to attack your body as if it were foreign. Kind of like an organ transplant reaction, but in reverse. Since he had his transplant he had had issues with his new immune system attacking his skin and his liver. Slowly, over the course of many months, well, years now, they were trying to wean him off the suppressants. The fewer immune suppressants he was taking the more his new immune system could work against the cancer. At any rate, the combination of therapies was doing something. His M-spike number for November was down to .2 g/dl.

Thanksgiving

The non-toxic Thanksgiving dinner we had planned went well. We arranged to get an heirloom, free-range, organic turkey. All of the potatoes, dairy products, vegetables, eggs and flour for the sides were organic. The only thing that wasn't organic was the corn meal for the cornbread stuffing, but it was Bob's Red Mill brand and, even though it wasn't one of their organic selections, it was probably better than a mainstream milled corn. Even our wine was safe—my brother hit up Pike & Western Wine Shop in Pike Place Market and picked up a variety of biodynamic wines, the product of natural wine growing topped with a little voodoo hippy magic. I'm not particularly fond of the biodynamic theory, but the wine was good and I couldn't complain.

The only potentially toxic snafu was when it came time to heat up the peas and onions from Cascadian Farms, a local farm that has a broad selection of organic frozen vegetables. We had put them in one of our glass storage bowls earlier in the day to defrost. These bowls are nothing too spectacular, just some product from Pyrex that comes with a plastic lid. Since the lids never touch the food, I wasn't too concerned about the plastic. Except, this time around, my brother heated up the peas in the microwave with the lid attached, which I didn't notice until it was pretty much done cooking and, at which point, I had a Non-Toxic Avenger hissy fit and gave him a tongue-lashing.

Although I knew that the lids were BPA-free, I still didn't know what kind of reaction they would have when put in the microwave and, while I didn't think they were dripping too much in the way of chemicals onto our peas, I still wasn't sure. As far as I could tell, the plastic lids were only to be used for fridge and freezer storage and not for heating. After digging around on the Pyrex website, I found the semi-magic words, "plastic lids are for microwave and storage use only." While this was encouraging to some degree, a lot of plastic products claim they are safe for the microwave. At that point, I was still in a bit of a quandary but there was no way to tell what, if any, impact there was. I could have taken the old "better safe than sorry" route, but I decided to eat the peas regardless.

Holiday lighting

My neighborhood goes absolutely crazy with holiday lighting. We didn't realize when we moved in five years earlier that there was a certain pressure to decorate. Our previous home was an old 1916 Craftsman-style house that didn't have any exterior electrical outlets so we never put up any outdoor Christmas decorations. A few of our neighbors did, but we would have to do some wiring work and that just wasn't going to happen. So, imagine our surprise when, as Christmas loomed in our new house, we started seeing the neighbors out in force. It starts Thanksgiving weekend, since most people have the extra time to spend setting up lights. If you don't have the time to do it yourself, you can hire people to do it for you. I had never seen advertisements for this sort of service before, but they start showing up at the end of November. Signs on poles, trucks with ads parked across the street from the entrance to our community. We didn't know we were moving into Holiday Central.

Our neighborhood is known in the Seattle area for its Christmas light displays and, over the years, it's become a destination. Part of our annual upkeep dues go to mounting a giant, lit, rotating Santa at the entrance and having someone dressed as Santa hand out candy canes on the weekends in December. I have yet to see the live Santa, but the rotating Santa is kind of fun in an old-fashioned sort of way. I didn't really believe the hype until the first year when I happened to look out the front window while I was talking on the telephone and I noticed that not only was there a stream of cars driving by, but there were tour buses as well. It was time to step up our game.

That first year, before I was really paying attention to our energy consumption, I got into a competition with our neighbors across the street. I initially put up a bunch of lights and then they one-upped me. I added more as I saw what others around the neighborhood were doing and the neighbors stepped it up a notch. This went back and forth until we had reached some serious illumination. I never stooped to the blow-up lit animals since I liked to keep the décor somewhat classic. Having said that, I can't deny that we blew the circuit at least once that year.

Since then, we've scaled it back considerably for a number of reasons. Primarily, it's a huge waste of resources, even if it is fun. Over the years we've replaced a lot of our string lighting with LED lights since, each year, LEDs have become cheaper and more readily available. Three years earlier, my husband had just been diagnosed with cancer and was in the hospital. When he did come home that November he was mostly immobile. I didn't have the energy, mental or otherwise, to put up much in the way of lights. Two years earlier my back went out right before Christmas and I never got around to putting up the lights. The previous year we waited too long and, by the time my husband decided we should put up some lights, the ground was frozen solid and we couldn't put up some of the lighting.

This year, however, I had a new plan. For the last 10 years or so, I've wanted to go to New Mexico during the holidays because I have a nasty fixation on *farolitos* or *luminarias* or whatever you want to call them. They're the paper bags filled with lights that are used to line pathways and rooflines. Back in the 1800s, bonfires (or *luminarias*) were used to light the way to the church for Christmas Mass. Today, that tradition continues during Christmastime. Since we weren't going to Santa Fe for Christmas, I thought we could bring New Mexico to Seattle. The issue is that paper bags and rain over the course of the four-week holiday lighting season wouldn't exactly work. So, I looked into electric *luminarias* and found what I wanted—reusable, plastic-based ones that would last the duration. I also wanted to hang outdoor chili pepper lights on the roof line and get a *chile ristra* or wreath for the door. My husband stopped me at the cow skull.

The problem with the chili pepper lights was that it would be very expensive to get the LED ones. Like, $100 more than the non-LED lights. So we decided to stick with our white LED lights for the roof line and get a few strands of the red LED chili pepper lights for accenting. Instead of getting a real *chile ristra*, we decided to go for one you could see in the night. In other words, one that lit up. We weren't going to have a giant light display this year, but it was going to be different.

One of the websites I visited when I was looking for lighting must have been a California business because it listed some additional warnings that other states don't need to put up. They had to do with lead in the wires of the lights. I hadn't thought at all about lead exposure when I was planning my Southwestern Holiday in the Northwest and it made me rethink what we were doing. Apparently, most Christmas lights have trace amounts of lead in the PVC wire. The State of California requires that Christmas lights with lead amounts above 300 ppm must be labeled with a lead warning, since the state's Scientific Advisory Board has determined that continuous close exposure could increase the risk of developing cancer. It is possible to find Christmas light sets with low-lead wire that does not exceed the 300 ppm threshold.

In the spirit of avoiding toxins, I went out and inspected the packaging for our LED lights from previous years to see if it had any information on it. Since it didn't, and I still suspected a trace amount of lead on those lights as well as any new ones, I determined it would probably be okay for a few reasons. The first was that I almost always wear gloves when putting up the lights, just because it's so cold out. I planned to immediately wash the gloves I used. The second reason was that, since the lights were outside (and frequently washed by the rain), my immediate exposure to both the lead and PVC wiring would be relatively insignificant.

While I was digging through the old box of lights I noticed an exceedingly strong telltale stench of vinyl. We have several strands of those rope lights, which are great for wrapping around trees but are nearly impossible to straighten out. No matter. I wasn't planning on using them, but after not having had them out for the last two holidays, I had forgotten how much the PVC rope lights smelled. And, since I was much more acutely aware of what that stench meant, I was wholeheartedly not interested in ever using them again. I checked out the new lights before I bought them to make sure they didn't have an excess of lead or other contaminants and deemed them semi-safe for the same reasons as I did our old lights. So, while we may not have had the hollyest or jollyest of lighting displays in our neighborhood, it was certainly one of the safest (no giant vinyl inflatables, although that inflatable cactus surely was tempting) and our decorations had a different spice to it. *Muy caliente!*

Off-gassing chess set

The weekend after Thanksgiving the family and I were out and about, picking up some holiday cheer. We ended up wandering into this fantastic little game shop in the Greenwood area of Seattle. They have more games there than you can shake a stick at, but not the classic Milton Bradley kind you can get at big-box toy stores. The store, Gary's Games and Hobbies, has a variety of interesting card games for kids as well as a myriad of more complicated games for adults. We picked up a few that Henry was interested in and both my husband and I were a bit surprised when he told us that he knew a little bit about chess.

Henry must have learned something about chess from school because he knew the names of some of the pieces. It's possible he picked it up somewhere else, like from a book or movie, but we can rarely tell since he generally doesn't self-report what's going on at school. In any case, he was interested in learning chess and, since my husband has been waiting for the day to teach him, it was another prime opportunity to pick up yet another chess set. I say "another" chess set because we already had several that Hank had purchased over the years since Henry was born. I knew of at least three we already owned, but that didn't stop him from buying another one in spite of my protests. I didn't think a $30 chess set was going to improve his chances of hooking Henry on the game any more than any of the other ones back at home.

Nevertheless, a new chess set was purchased, this time with heavier pieces and a flexible board. Unfortunately, when he took the game out of the box and went to set it up he didn't notice what the chess board was made out of. I immediately noticed it because the dining room table smelled like someone had unrolled an inflatable raft on the table. It was made with PVC—the same incriminating, off-gassing spectacle that lines showers, binders and raincoats nationwide. The same material that can contain phthalates, lead and cadmium, and can be toxic to a child's health.

I had my second Thanksgiving weekend Non-Toxic Avenger hissy fit and immediately rolled the "board" back up and put it back in its box to off-gas a little more slowly and, preferably, somewhere else. Like the basement closet. I then implored my husband to use one of the other chess boards we had on hand. It took a few minutes to locate an appropriate wood one, but he managed to find it just fine. And the kids were able to start their long fixation with the game without breathing in a load of chemicals to scramble their hardworking minds in the process.

Oh! Christmas tree

For years, my husband and I had purchased real trees for our Christmas tree. I had grown up with a plastic, fake tree, a huge behemoth that had color-coded limbs and took far too much time to assemble. When I first met my husband in college 20 years ago, the idea of an actual tree for Christmas was a foreign concept. My mom was always against it, probably for cost issues, but mainly because I think having to deal with buying and transporting it, watering it and getting rid of it was too much of a pain. We also heard the oft-employed excuse about her allergies that pretty much shut down any arguing for a real tree. When my husband (then boyfriend) suggested getting a real tree for Christmas I thought it was going to be a disaster, having been indoctrinated all those years against them. When we started bringing them home I hated the needle-drop issue but loved the smell and the tradition of going and picking one out. We carried on like this for over 10 years or so and the thought of getting a fake tree never even crossed my mind. Until my husband got sick.

One of the benefits of having a fake tree is that it comes apart. And, for someone such as myself who routinely has a bad back, the convenience of separating it into easy-to-carry pieces was quite alluring. The first Christmas after my husband's diagnosis, when he was pretty much bedbound and could barely walk, I decided that pursuing an LED-lit fake tree (floor model, with deep discount) wasn't such a bad idea after all. You just flip open the stand, insert a few pieces, plug it in *et voilà!* Easy-squeezy Christmas tree. Most people who saw it thought it was real—it didn't have that "fake tree" look screaming from its branches. However, under all that ease and handsome good looks lurked something I knowingly took into my home—the knowledge that my tree was made in China, out of PVC and, undoubtedly, a lot of lead.

The issue with fake Christmas trees and their PVC content is not too different than the issue with PVCs in general. Much like a shower curtain, they shed chemicals like phthalates, cadmium and other volatile organic compounds. And, since my kids tend to sit near the tree for the month that it's up, that's a lot of exposure. Add to the fact that it's also made out of lead and you have a very bad combination. The Children's Health Environmental Coalition warns that fake trees "may shed lead-laced dust, which may cover branches or shower gifts and the floor below the tree."[1] And shower the kids who are sitting under the tree staring at the lights in anticipation.

I ignored this fact the following year when my husband was post-transplant and incredibly weak. Again, I could easily do the fake tree myself rather than having to haul a real tree into the house alone. The next year after that our fake tree was up yet again, but we weren't around much. We ended up putting up the tree late and then were out of town for almost the entirety of Christmas break. The year of this book project, however, particularly with the non-toxic action in play, there was no excuse and our fake tree stayed (somewhat) safely bagged in the basement. In spite of not wanting to spend money on a new tree when we already had one, I knew it was the right thing to do. Having a bunch of holiday dollars at our local nursery didn't exactly hurt so we went off to check out their reindeer and camels on Thanksgiving weekend and picked up our Christmas tree.

Getting orthopedic

After Thanksgiving, I finally went in to see the podiatrist about the continuing problems I was having with the sesamoiditis pain in my left foot. The last time I had gone in to get it checked out, the podiatrist had suggested that I get custom orthotics to help protect that area of my foot so it could heal. Because the pain had been going on and off for almost a year by this point it was worth the energy and expense of getting orthotics. The podiatrist I met with this time was great. We went over my biomechanical issues (high arch, tibial angle and inflexibility) and chit-chatted while he cast my feet. He was very interested in this book and what I had found out so far. Having a degree in engineering (in addition to an MD) he mentioned that he was curious about the health effects of electromagnetic and other unseen and unheard waves constantly bombarding us.

Aside from talking toxins, we also discussed my treatment options and he handed me a list of recommended shoes that would help with my healing. I had taken with me my walking and running shoes as well as my old orthotics that I used to use for running to help control the over-pronation, or "rolling in," my feet tend to do. My current walking shoes were determined to be too soft for my problems, but my running shoes were stable enough. On the list were some shoes with a rocker sole that he highlighted as being best for my current foot condition.

He circled the Dansko shoes, which I had but which tended to aggravate my problems because of the hard insole. The other shoe he circled as recommended was the Skechers Shape-ups, those funny-looking round-bottomed shoes that allegedly help firm up your calves and butt. I certainly couldn't argue against any assistance there and any extra foot comfort would be appreciated as well. I did a little recon online to learn more about them, as I do with pretty much everything. I had a couple different options with the shoes — it turned out there were a lot more styles of them available than I realized.

Unfortunately, the majority of the ones designed for walking had an antibacterial treatment, which I expected to be some chemical variant of triclosan. Triclosan is one of those insidious chemicals that shows up in more products than I care to imagine. It's not just a mainstay in antibacterial soaps, but also makes an appearance in everything from toothpaste to toys to cosmetics. It has been strongly linked to endocrine abnormalities, immune-system weakening and cancer. Like other persistent organic pollutants, this one doesn't go away — it gets stored in your body. While it was unlikely that I would be absorbing much of the chemical through my shoes, I didn't want any exposure to it, however small.

The one style of Sketcher rocker-sole shoe that I had my eye on, mostly because it was not as obvious as the others, not only didn't claim to have the antibacterial coating, it also sported a "Roll Control" technology to help with over-pronation. It sounded just like what the doctor ordered. I went out and purchased a pair of the ones geared more for running and didn't see any sign on the material listing that came with them of an antibacterial coating. Between the shoes and the orthotics, I was hopeful that I would be able to get rid of the sesamoiditis once and for all.

CFLs and dirty electricity

When my podiatrist mentioned that he had always been concerned about the effects of electric and magnetic frequencies (EMFs) emitted by radio and cell phone towers, not to mention appliances and other electronics, I asked if he had heard about the study done on the correlation between the health of diabetics and the kinds of dirty electricity generated by energy-saving electronics and compact fluorescent lights (CFLs).[2] He hadn't, which wasn't too surprising, as the study was small. The authors of the study concluded that, in an environment free of EMFs, Type 1 diabetics needed less insulin and Type 2 diabetics had lower blood glucose levels. The researchers also noted that diabetes testing done in a high-EMF environment could lead to false positives. While the research done on diabetics so far has been claimed by other researchers to be somewhat dubious, I certainly would like to see some more work done to either confirm or dispel this theory.

Because most of us are completely unaware of the constant bombardment of low- and high-level frequencies being generated all around us from our microwaves to our cordless and cell phones, little thought or attention is paid to them. More recently has been the concern about the type of electricity generated from CFL bulbs and other energy-saving devices. The issue is that high-frequency voltage transients, aka "dirty electricity," are a by-product of energy-efficient electronics and appliances. These energy-efficient electronics reduce the amount of electricity they use by chopping up the voltage. In doing so, they create a wildly fluctuating electromagnetic field that not only radiates into the immediate environment but can also back up along your wiring all the way back to the utility, hitting every energy customer in between. So, even if you unplug all of your electronics and are "going Amish" at home, your distant neighbor could be impacting you with dirty electricity from afar, unless you've unplugged yourself from the grid.

Dr. Olle Johansson, a Swedish neuroscientist, claims that "the human body, whose cells, nerves and organs function with electrical impulse, have [*sic*] difficulty adapting to 60-Hertz cycles, let alone transient high frequencies that last milliseconds. We are dealing with amplitude-modulated or pulsed microwaves in the 2.45 Ghz range (or nearby), in a form that has only been around to any extent for the last 10–15 years. Compared to the natural background fields, in which living cells have developed during the last 3.8 billion years, these electromagnetic fields are actually very,

very strong. It is thus wrong to believe that evolution has furnished us with a safety protection shielding layer against such WLAN (wireless local area network) signals. It has not."[3]

In doing the research on this for a blog post, I ran across some suggestions for how to reduce one's exposure to dirty electricity. Suggestions from *Prevention* magazine included such things as reducing exposure to wireless Internet, getting rid of dimmer switches, limiting CFLs, using a landline phone rather than a cordless phone, avoiding Bluetooth headsets, avoiding cell phones when the signal is low, charging your laptop when it's not on your lap and unplugging everything when you aren't using it.[4] As part of this project I had to consider how much the whole concept of "dirty electricity" was really impacting me and whether or not it could be classified as being an environmental toxin. Was it worth including in the book and doing something about it, particularly in light of the fact that there really wasn't much hard data on the studies done so far?

As with chemical toxicants, we don't see a direct cause and effect with EMFs, although several studies suggest potential mayhem. Based on just my gut feeling on the matter, I decided to do a few things to reduce my exposure. Primarily this included really getting my butt in gear in not just turning off electronics and appliances when not in use, but unplugging them altogether. A plugged-in appliance in many cases draws electricity regardless of whether or not you are actively using it and is probably doing its volt-chopping magic anyway.

I rarely use a cell phone, so I wasn't too concerned about that particular piece of equipment. I generally only use it for emergencies. However, since my cell phone was on its last legs (it was at least eight years old), I took note that, if I ever needed a new one, the Environmental Working Group had a webpage listing the cell phones that emit the least amount of radiation.[5] My husband and I checked the site to see how his cell phone fared, as he uses his a lot more than I do mine, and it didn't rank very well at all. It was a new Android phone and it was unlikely he'd be swapping it out anytime soon, so the best thing he could do was to use a headset when he talked on it and only use it when he's got a decent signal. If you have a low signal the phone has to work harder (meaning sending out more EMFs) trying to get a signal.

As for our microwave, I had been ambivalent about it off and on for a while. I punted the decision to get rid of it entirely due to its utility and energy savings and satisfied myself by finding a way to conveniently unplug it between uses to keep down the amount of EMFs emanating from it. Additionally, I went around the house, unplugging things not in use and only plugging them in when they were needed. It was additional work to do so, but really not that inconvenient—just a new learned behavior.

The biggest potential issue was really with my laptop for two reasons. Since I sat with it on my lap for an extended number of hours every day, I was being exposed to not just EMFs from the machine itself, particularly when it was charging, but also from the Wi-Fi signal that I was constantly using. And not just from our own Wi-Fi signal, but also from all those hotspots in the neighborhood and pretty much everywhere I went that was in an urban setting. I started using as much battery power as possible when I used it but, inevitably, I had to plug it in when it ran low after a few hours. At least it would reduce some of the exposure. I looked into getting a pad that you place under your laptop and that allegedly blocks up to 100% of the EMFs generated and disperses the heat generated. I already used a product called the Laplander that provided heat protection and a cushion, but the EMFs were not blocked. I decided to purchase a HaraPad Elite. According to their website, it blocks 100% of the EMFs by acting as a ground to the circulating EMFs. It essentially catches the stray electromagnetic field and returns it safely to the laptop to complete the circuit.

The second thing I did with my laptop was to disable the wireless connection when I didn't absolutely need it. This helped out twofold. It removed the Wi-Fi signal from my laptop (although that's not to say I wasn't still being bombarded by the Wi-Fi hotspots surrounding my home and elsewhere for that matter) and it reduced the distraction from looking at websites on the Internet. Working on a computer is difficult when it comes to easy distractions and I'm easily distracted. Constant access to email, the Internet and Facebook usually makes for a dangerous combination and low productivity. Turning off the Wi-Fi required more planning when I was doing Internet research, but that just meant I needed to have the appropriate document open online before I shut it down. And cranking it back up for an emergent need wasn't too difficult. Being cut off forced me to concentrate on my writing tasks. However, since so much of what I do and write on my blog and for this book required Internet access for reference, it ended up affecting my productivity almost as much as being connected. An alternative would have been to work on an actual LAN connection with the Wi-Fi off, but by doing so I would be sitting closer to far more electronics than by working upstairs, remotely, away from the computer hub of activity.

CFL bulbs are known to emit dirty electricity and are also known to trigger migraines, dizziness and loss of focus. I've had problems with fluorescent lighting in stores and other public spaces triggering migraines for years. Because of the potential for migraines and the fact that I needed as much focus as I could get, I decided to remove the CFL bulbs we had in the house and either replaced them with LED bulbs where I could or went back to incandescent ones elsewhere. As much as I was a huge proponent of saving electricity where possible, there were just too many emerging issues with CFLs in regards to mercury and their disposal. Add to that the UV radiation, frequency and dirty electricity generated by these new bulbs, as well as the compelling argument that LED bulbs didn't have the same issues, and it just didn't make sense to me to continue using CFLs. Different problems may emerge in the future with LEDs as they become more prevalent but, in the meantime, I made the decision to stick with the old-fashioned bulbs and LEDs.

Happy pits

I finally did it! I made a deodorant concoction that worked at keeping me stink-free in spite of exercising and has on occasion lasted two days when a shower just didn't make it into the day. Not only that, but my armpits weren't irritated and, more importantly, they didn't turn brown and my armpit skin didn't thicken up and slough off in sheets. I found this last mixture so gentle and effective that I could use it every day. I no longer even bothered using the Crystal deodorant and only sporadically used the unscented Ban Roll-On when I needed an actual antiperspirant, which was relatively rare.

I ended up nixing the baking soda altogether because it left such a grit to the mixture that all day long the rubbing was painful. My latest trial deodorant recipe consisted of two tablespoons each of organic coconut oil and cocoa butter, with about 2 teaspoons of corn starch. I also added in some essential oils to give it some "flavor" (vanilla and sandalwood) and ended up with some mighty fine chocolate cookie–smelling happy pits.

Getting bloody

Almost four years ago I switched what I was using during my menstrual period to a product that was more sustainable. Since the average woman generates about 350 pounds of waste from menstrual products during her lifetime — enough to fill an entire dump truck — it's something that needs to be taken seriously. The National Women's Health Network estimates that, in the U.S. alone, more than 12 billion pads and 7 million tampons are disposed of every year. That's a tremendous amount of garbage and one that I didn't want to contribute to anymore.

Aside from the garbage issue, however, I also wanted to reduce my exposure to toxins. The cotton in conventional menstrual products is bleached with chlorine which produces dioxin. Dioxin is the main ingredient in Agent Orange and is linked to cancer, reproductive problems, disruption of regulatory hormones and immune system damage. Most conventional products (not organic or "natural") also have synthetic fragrances as well as trace amounts of aluminum. None of which I really wanted my nether regions directly exposed to.

Because of this, I switched to a medical-grade silicone reusable menstrual cup called the DivaCup, which essentially replaces tampons. The risk of toxic shock syndrome is relatively nil and, once you get the hang of it, it's very convenient and it works extremely well for most women. I only need to empty and clean it twice a day when in use and I consider it to be one of the greatest inventions known to womankind. I often joke on my blog that if I were going to take one thing with me to a deserted island it would be my DivaCup.

When I first heard of these reusable cup things, I thought it was a joke or, at the very least, something that couldn't possibly be effective. I figured that it was some product cooked up by the same women who crotchet their own tampons. At first, it took about a month to really figure out how to use it properly but now I love it. Not just because it saves me money and reduces my waste considerably but also because it makes my period easier. It's not really something I think about anymore since there is so much less hassle.

I didn't really do anything different for this project regarding what I was using for my period since I was already using something non-toxic. But it did remind me that before, when I was using conventional products, I was being exposed to some fairly unsavory potential toxins. As with most other toxin exposures, it is difficult to calculate out the true risk with them, but with my current product it's not something I need to think about. Ever again.

Getting sick from medications

Unlike my husband, who still is on a variety of daily medications (his pill organizer is pretty much a 5 × 7 pill pack dispensary), I don't take anything besides the occasional ibuprofen for cramps or muscle pain and the every-once-in-a-while aspirin if I get a migraine. I limit my usage as much as possible but the last time I took an ibuprofen I did take notice that, for some reason, the one I had on hand was coated in a variety of strange, artificial colors ranging from burgundy to neon orange. It was bad enough I was taking a medication that was hard on my liver, so I went in search of white, uncolored ibuprofen. The aspirin, on the other hand, was uncoated and white so there wasn't an issue there. The other fillers in my plain aspirin were relatively minimal so I wasn't too worried about what I was using in regards to my aspirin usage. The ibuprofen was another story and it wasn't just the coloring.

As I was researching phthalates, I discovered that they were also found in medications where they were used as an inactive ingredient to produce enteric coatings, otherwise known as the coating that protects your stomach.[6] Since my aspirin wasn't enteric-coated it wasn't a problem, but I made sure my newly purchased white ibuprofen didn't have a coating as well, which was harder than it sounds. Most products on the market have a cellulose coating and/or contain polyethylene glycol (PEG). Furthermore, brand names like Advil can contain parabens and sodium lauryl sulfate (SLS), Motrin has artificial colors and PEGs, and generic names brands have artificial colors and PEGs and cellulose coatings, so it took a bit of looking around to find a product that didn't contain a bunch of other unwanted inactive ingredients. Trying to find one that wasn't colored or coated was difficult. I settled on getting an uncolored brand and just tried to limit my usage as much as I could.

Vitamin supplements have similar problems with inactive ingredients, mostly related to artificial colors and flavors. Earlier in the year we had switched all of our vitamins to "natural" brands that used food sources (like annatto and beets) for coloring in the vitamins and didn't contain any artificial fillers. Even so, I went back and made sure other unwanted ingredients weren't slipping into our diet by way of vitamins.

Washing it all away

A few years prior to this project we had switched over from a heavily fragranced, artificially colored and petroleum-based laundry detergent to something a little more skin- and earth-friendly. It took a while to find a brand that worked well enough to supplant a more robust commercial detergent like Tide, but we found it (Biokleen Laundry Powder) and haven't looked back since. When we travel we oftentimes get stuck using commercial brands and I'm reminded of how much they stink, being full of artificial fragrances and bleaching agents.

We faced the same ordeal with dishwashing detergents. We tried a ton of them until we found one that worked just as well as Cascade or Electrosol, but without the phosphates, fragrance, petroleum, bleach and other nasty chemicals. As mentioned earlier, our favorite machine-dishwashing detergent of choice became Ecover Dishwasher Tablets. For hand-dishwashing we used Planet Ultra Dishwashing Liquid. Planet was great in that it also doubled as a fruit and vegetable wash and, since it didn't have any added fragrance or dyes and was gentle, we could pretty much use it for anything, even as bubble bath or a pet shampoo if we were so inclined. More importantly it worked well. It didn't cut through grease as well as something like Dawn, but we just needed to employ a little more elbow grease to the actual grease. And, really, we rarely had something that greasy that we need a more caustic cleaning fluid. And, if we did, we added in some Bon Ami for non-toxic scrubbing.

While the Ecover had added fragrance listed in the ingredients, I couldn't really smell anything when we ran the dishwasher. It didn't have that pungent chlorine and fragrance odor but that didn't mean that it wasn't off-gassing phthalates. So I did a little digging about the fragrance ingredients. Being a Belgian company, Ecover follows tighter standards than U.S. companies. The material safety data sheet for the dishwasher tablets stated, "does not contain any ingredients known to be mutagenic, carcinogenic, teratogenic or reproduction toxic" and "Ecover products do not contain any bioaccumulating raw materials and no PCM or nitromusk perfume components."[7] After a bit more searching, the fragrance turned out to be citrus based. Limonene in fact.

There are some issues with limonene, although I haven't been throwing out products if they contain it since it's generally used as a scent ingredient and is a solvent that occurs naturally in the rind of citrus fruit. According to the Skin Deep website, when exposed to sunlight or air limonene can degrade to various oxidation products which, in turn, can be a skin and respiratory irritant. The same thing can probably be said anytime I ate an orange, so suffice it to say, I concluded that the Ecover tablets were "safe" enough.

Coffee log

I love a good roaring fire and, even though it doesn't produce much heat in our household because we have an open fireplace, I still like to burn a log every now and again, especially during the holidays. The problem with burning wood in a fireplace that isn't an actual wood-burning stove that regulates the amount of particulate matter is that the smoke can be harmful to breathe in. The average person should be concerned about lighting a fire in an open fireplace if someone in the house has asthma or chronic obstructive pulmonary disease (COPD) or some other lung problem. Burning wood in a nonEPA-certified woodstove or fireplace can release carbon monoxide, nitrogen oxides, hydrocarbons, formaldehyde, dioxins, volatile organic compounds (such as benzene) and furans. The latter three are known carcinogens. In our family, we don't like burning wood and we especially don't like burning regular fire logs because of the questionable materials in them.

Over the last couple of years, more natural fire logs have come on the market. More recently, I had been getting emails about a fire log product made out of waxed cardboard. And while a waxed cardboard product like Enviro-Log burns 30–40% cleaner with lower particulate matter emissions than firewood and is better than a traditional fire log as far as emissions go, it's still not what I wanted to be breathing in. It was certainly better than a traditional fire log in that it used resources that would otherwise be sent to the landfill, but the wax from the cardboard was still petroleum-based and it would be no better than burning paraffin candles as far as toxins go.

If we wanted to burn something in the fireplace, we would use the product we've used for the last several years in spite of the desire to throw on a real piece of wood. That product is the Java-Log from Pine Mountain. The Java-Log emits up to 78% less carbon monoxide and 66% less creosote than regular wood. It uses renewable natural-based waxes and, most importantly, it diverts a ton of used coffee grounds from the waste stream. However, when I went to the EPA website and saw the comparisons for emissions between Java-Log and other natural fire logs, I was extremely surprised. Out of the five different logs tested, the emission rate for the Java-Log fell in the middle, with the Northland and the Pine Mountain Superlog emitting less carbon monoxide. On the emission rate for particulate matter, Java-Log came in second after Northland (with the Java-Log coming in at 8 $PM_{2.5}$/[g/hr] versus 60 for cordwood). It was much higher than the rest in aluminum, copper, zinc, manganese and phosphorus but relatively low in lead and mercury.

Of all the fire logs studied it looked like, overall, the best as far as emissions went was the Northland Firelog with the Superlog edging out the Java-Log by a hair. If we wanted to burn a fire log we would still go with the Java-Log because the differential wasn't that big overall, and because the environmental impact of the Java-Log was less than that of the other two options. Plus, we already had some Java-Logs and the other two brands were difficult to find.[8] By the end of the project we ended up burning exactly zero fire logs altogether, so it became a complete non-issue.

The not-so-zen yoga mat

With my new rocker sole shoes and an increase in activity, I started to stretch a lot more. Or, rather, I *needed* to stretch a whole lot more. I have, for almost 20 years, been extremely inflexible. I don't know exactly when that started but it was sometime around the time I started running in my early 20s. With the increase in muscle came a decrease in flexibility in spite of all the stretching I felt like I was doing. I've known people who rarely stretch, but are much more flexible than I am and I've never quite been able to figure out why. My inflexibility causes me a lot of problems, most notably with my knees when I am running (which I don't really do anymore because of the foot issues) and most painfully with my back. My tight calves, hamstrings, hip flexors and a number of other lower body muscles and tendons all end up pulling on my back, causing me a lot of problems with back spasms and strains. If I stay on top of stretching and make sure I do it every day, then I can keep most of my back pain at bay. Even if I skip one day, I'm setting myself up for pain later.

With the increase in exercise I really needed to stretch twice a day and by that I mean a combination of classic running stretches as well as yoga. The problem with yoga is that most yoga mats are made out of or are backed with PVC. We had three yoga mats in the house because the kids were big into imitating my yoga practice for a while there. The mats didn't get a tremendous amount of use, but they were still present, off-gassing dangerous chemicals (like phthalates, lead and cadmium) into our rooms.

If I stretched in the living room, there was enough padding under the rug that I didn't need a mat. However, if I wanted to do anything that required a sticky mat, it was an issue because I slipped on the rug. Fortunately, there are yoga mats that are made out of non-toxic thermoplastic elastomer (TPE), rather than PVC.[9] If I wanted to take a yoga class, I could bring my own non-PVC mat, but I'd still be in a room full of people using, most likely, PVC mats. All that deep-breathing just meant that I'd be deep-breathing in a room full of PVC particulates. I hated to do it, but I donated all three of our yoga mats. Since I still needed at least one mat in the house, I ordered a TPE-based mat. The one really nice thing about the new mat was the fact that it didn't have that "new mat" smell.

Body art

In 2004, the American Environmental Safety Institute filed a law-suit against a half dozen or so tattoo ink pigment manufacturers, claiming they failed to warn California residents about exposure to hazardous materials in their inks. The lead content found in the ink needed for a medium-sized tattoo could potentially contain between 1 and 23 micrograms of lead, which is considerably more than the 0.5 microgram per day recommended limit. Some inks also contained metals such as aluminum, arsenic, mercury and chromium in addition to lead. The heavy metals are used to give the pigments their permanent color, not unlike other artist paints, and the type of metal depends mostly on the color pigment as well as the manufacturer.[10]

Considering that one in four adults in the U.S. has at least one tattoo, with many of them sporting quite a few, this is an issue that really needs more widespread education on the potential risks of toxicity. I have two tattoos of small to medium size. I have no interest in getting them removed even though it would make sense since I am exposed to the metals from the pigments. However, there are a few issues with laser tattoo removal. The first issue is that additional chemicals are used on the skin to reduce the surface temperature so your skin doesn't scar. The more commonly used chemical is tetrafluoroethane, which is a very toxic greenhouse gas. The alternative, which is considered to be more "green," is a carbon dioxide spray, or rather, a dry ice spray which is better for your skin and the ozone layer.[11]

The big issue with laser tattoo removal is that, when you break down the pigments into small particles, the body has to do something with them. Research done at the National Center for Toxicological Research (NCTR) has been studying how tattoo ink breaks down in your body either from exposure to sunlight or natural degradation and the main question to be answered is, where does the pigment go? Is it broken down by enzymes or metabolized? In at least one study, researchers found that some pigment migrates from the tattoo site to the body's lymph nodes.[12] Considering that chemists at the NCTR identified low levels of carcinogens in tattoo ink, what kind of health impact is there in having a tattoo? And, if this is occurring under the normal lifetime of a tattoo, what happens when you try to remove it?

German scientists have shown that, after laser irradiation during removal, the concentrations of toxic molecules from red and yellow tattoo inks increased up to 70-fold.[13] Heat on the pigment triggers a chemical reaction that generates mutation-inducing and carcinogenic breakdown products that get reabsorbed by the body. One last point on tattoos and metals—the FDA warns that patients about to undergo an MRI should let the technician know they have a tattoo because it can swell or burn, most likely from the metals in the pigments.[14] This last factoid was something to keep in mind if I had to go in to the neurologist for that MRI in case the numbness and tingling reoccurred in my arms and legs.

Tingle time

A few weeks after I started experiencing the numbness and tingling in my arms and legs in August I started taking some supplements, mostly Vitamin B12 and Vitamin D3 because I tested low for both. Several weeks after I began the supplements the symptoms totally went away. At the time, I never did figure out what caused them and I never did find out why they went away. I did try challenging my sunscreen theory since the sunscreen was the only new thing that I was exposed to before the tingling began. I used this new sunscreen again off and on right before my initial body burden lab testing but I never experienced any renewed numbness and tingling. So, I scratched that off my list of potential aggravators.

When I was looking into some of the results from my lab tests and saw that certain solvents can cause tingling and muscle pain, it reminded me of the fact that I had been doing a blog experiment with a solvent the weeks before I started having the tingling, numbness and muscle pain problem. This made me wonder whether or not this experiment was the cause of what I was feeling. I didn't really want to test this new theory because I didn't want to recreate the symptoms since they were so annoying and somewhat painful. It took a few months for me to be willing to challenge this theory as well.

Back in August I was already experimenting with reducing our exposure to chemical cleaners when I ran across a product that removed soap scum without any hazardous chemicals. It was essentially a stone, kind of like pumice but not as abrasive, that you use with water to scrub off the soap scum. With a little elbow grease, it was quite effective on our shower and I wrote a blog post about it. Some readers warned me that those types of scrubbers can scratch the tiles on your shower, thereby inviting more mold growth and making soap scum even harder to remove in the future. I didn't know how much truth there was to the risks of using this particular product but while I was doing some more research on it someone suggested using rubbing alcohol to remove soap scum.

I figured (back then) that rubbing alcohol was safer to use than something like Scrubbing Bubbles and can be applied to the skin, so it must be safe to use. I had applied more isopropyl rubbing alcohol than I care to remember to my husband's chest when he had a Hickman catheter for more than a year after his transplants. Of course, I used to wear rubber gloves when I did this. This time around, I didn't bother. Mostly because I had spontaneously decided, right before going in the shower, to give it a try and I didn't want to get suited up with gloves. So, I loaded up a sponge with rubbing alcohol and went to work. And, by gum, the soap scum came off like crazy. It was almost miraculous and I probably spent far too much time scrubbing and exposing myself to rubbing alcohol than I should have.

Now, of course, I realize that it worked because rubbing alcohol is considered to be a solvent. A solvent that magically removes soap scum with a single swipe and, just maybe, also causes tingling and muscle pain. It was the only other thing that potentially could have been causing the problems. It wasn't until after Thanksgiving that I decided to give it another whirl, this time wearing gloves, so the experiment wasn't exactly complete. But the shower door needed a good soap scum removal and I figured I'd try just exposing myself to the fumes which were, after months of living without anything perfumed or fragranced, noxious to say the least and made me doubt my intelligence. Even though I didn't experience any tingling or numbness, at least with that type of exposure, the rubbing alcohol did clean the shower door nicely.

Since the symptoms were so fleeting I stopped worrying about having an underlying health problem. My mom had also been experiencing a lot of numbness and tingling in her legs and feet and finally went and got checked out not too soon after I started having problems. She thought that maybe she too had low Vitamin B12 or Vitamin D and maybe that was contributing to her symptoms. My mom has other issues that I don't have, though, namely weakness in the muscles that lift your feet. She was preliminarily diagnosed with a neuromuscular degenerative disease that was genetic in nature, meaning that I had a high probability of having it too. Given the fact that my symptoms went away, whether or not by nutritional supplementation or by less exposure to some neurotoxin, I can't say for sure if they were early signs of this disease as well. But knowing I might have a predisposition to this other disorder is certainly something I needed to be aware of as I get older or if the problems return.

Lab results unearthed!

In early December I finally got the lab results back for the chlorinated pesticides, PCBs and volatile solvents combined body burden tests that I had done months earlier. It turned out the lab results were sent to the wrong doctor's inbox, but they were able to get the lab, Metametrix, to fax over another copy of the test results.

The first testing group, chlorinated pesticides, tested for the more commonly known pesticides like DDT/DDE, oxychlordane, mirex, dieldrin and hexachlorobenzene. Chlorinated pesticides are persistent in the environment, meaning that they don't go away, and they bioaccumulate (or build-up) in our bodies, particularly in our organs and fat. These chemicals are easily passed to infants through breastfeeding and through the placenta. Most ingestion of chlorinated pesticides comes through food as pesticide residue as well as from drinking water since the chemicals can leach through the soil and into drinking water.

These particular toxicants affect the nervous tissue and muscle membranes. They can result in chronic neurological problems and can cause difficulties with learning and memory. They have also been shown to cause diabetes, heart disease, certain cancers and other health issues.[15] They really are a nasty group of chemicals particularly since they just don't seem to want to go away. DDT, dieldrin and mirex, for example, have been banned from use in the United States since the 1970s but, since they are chemicals that are persistent organic pollutants in the environment, babies born today are still at risk of exposure.

In animal products, particularly the fattier cuts as well as high-fat butter, cheese and whole milk, the toxins end up accumulating as higher concentrations as you go up the food chain. This is known as biomagnification. So, all the chlorinated pesticides and fungicides ingested by the cow, whose milk you are currently drinking, are getting passed on to you. That's why eating organic dairy and meat is so important. And that's why I was ecstatic to find out that I only had minor detectable levels of DDE (a metabolite, or breakdown product, of DDT) with all other pesticides being undetectable. This is great news because of the difficulty in ridding one's body of these accumulating toxins that get trapped in fat. There's not much I can do to prevent future exposure to most of these banned pesticides, but there are still others in use, so continuing to eat organic can only help keep those numbers low. As for ridding my body of what I do have, a detox program can help with that.

How do my results stack up against others' results? The only chlorinated pesticide that was detectable was DDE.

Deanna Duke's results
0.36 ppb in serum
95th percentile (ppb): 12.10
Lipid adjusted results: 71.9 ng/g lipid
95th percentile (ng/g lipid): 1,860

EWG/Commonweal results are based on individual DDE chemical components versus the grouping done by Metametrix and aren't comparable.

The next set of tests were all related to the PCBs, or polychlorinated biphenyls, and tested for eight common ones, both dioxin-like and nondioxin-like. Banned from use in 1979, these commonly used lubricants and coolants don't break down in the environment and continue to leach into the soil and groundwater from hazardous-waste sites and landfills. Like the chlorinated pesticides, PCBs are stored in fatty tissues and bioaccumulate over a person's lifetime. They are shown to cause health problems with neurobehavioral and immune-system development, resulting in the possibility of psychomotor and behavioral problems, obesity and even some cancers.[16]

Again, I was overjoyed to find out that all eight PCBs tested for were undetectable in my labs. This isn't to say that I didn't have any PCBs or DDT, etc., in my body, it just means they weren't circulating around in my bloodstream in detectable levels. As mentioned earlier, the only truly definitive method of testing would be a fat biopsy.

Last, but not least, was the volatile solvents panel of tests which included such nasties as benzene, ethylbenzene, m,p-xylene, styrene, toluene, hexane, 2-methylpentane and 3-methylpentane. Chronic exposure to volatile solvents can cause damage to your central nervous system and your liver and kidneys. Benzene can have serious effects on the hematological system (how your body makes blood) and is a recognized human carcinogen. It is one of the suspected carcinogens that causes multiple myeloma, the type of bone marrow cancer my husband has.

Other solvents can cause loss of coordination, vision problems, muscle pain and tingling. Solvents, in general, are very damaging to bone marrow and are associated with bone marrow cancers, immune disorders, chronic neurological problems and infertility. Unlike the other contaminants like DDT and PCBs, most of these solvents are still in use today and, unfortunately, in large quantities. Annual production of these solvents in the United States numbers in the tens of billions of pounds. Exposure generally occurs from air and water as well as by inhaling or ingesting car exhaust, paints, glues, adhesives and paint thinners.[17]

I had minor detectable levels of ethylbenzene, hexane, 2-methyl-pentane, 3-methylpentane and isooctane. All other volatile solvents were undetectable. Except for m,p-xylene, wherein I had a "significant elevation" (above the 95th percentile). This last one freaked me out a bit until I remembered that Chanel nail polish. While styrene was the only solvent listed on the ingredients, I wouldn't be too surprised if there were some xylenes in the product as well. Final testing (without using any nasty nail polish) will be the true test as to my general exposure to this solvent.

It's important to point out that the human body is efficient at mostly processing out the xylene solvents within about 48 hours. Styrene takes even less time. What kind of residual amount accumulates in the body fat and organs is not readily known but the main issue is the chronic exposure. If such high levels are obtained from mere nail polish, and if one tends to use nail polish on a weekly basis, those bloodstream levels of solvents are going to be kept at a high level day after day. That is also not to mention the risk to nail artists who are breathing in these fumes all day, every day.

The same risk exists for painters who work with lacquers and paint thinners, mechanics who inhale car exhaust in semi-contained areas and a number of other people, including artists working with solvents and oil paints. At best, they will experience headaches, brain fog, fatigue, chronic infections and eye and skin irritation. At worst, they are exposing themselves to B-cell malignancies, leukemia, muscle weakness, Parkinson's and renal damage.

When our house was painted the spring before I started working on this book I went out of my way to make sure the paint we used on the house was as "Earth-friendly" as possible. However, that message didn't quite get across when it came to the door. Our painter used a lacquer that smelled horrifically strong. If I stayed in the house for more than a few minutes I felt really confused and in a fog. At first I thought I was just imagining the problems, but after reading about the health effects of these chemicals, I'm fairly sure I wasn't making up the symptoms I was experiencing.

Throw your watch away

Fremont is a Seattle neighborhood quite close to where we live. It used to be a hub of counterculture. Not only does it sport a giant Lenin statue on the main street (which is currently for sale if you have $250k and are interested) but it also bears signs instructing residents and visitors to "Throw your watch away." Well, I did just that. I didn't *actually* throw out my watch, but I went back to my possibly toxic watch. After not being able to see the numbers on the non-toxic watch face for months, the final straw was when I accidentally got the watchband slightly wet when Henry was in the bath. While the watch is allegedly water resistant, the band certainly is not and having a soaking wet organic cotton watchband was no fun. But that was not reason enough to throw out the watch.

When I woke up the next morning, I put on the watch with the now dry watchband and noticed that the watch face made me think of the scene from *Pulp Fiction* with Christopher Walken. The one where his character explains that the watch (which is visibly steamed up) had survived being confiscated by being stored up two people's hindquarters for years during the Vietnam War. In any case, the watch face eventually dried out after a couple of days and I went back to wearing it. But that still didn't resolve the issue that I couldn't make out half the numbers most of the time.

It wasn't until I made a grave error in calendar dates that I decided enough was enough. I rely heavily on my watch, rather than a calendar, to remind me what date it is, otherwise I'm relatively clueless. Since I couldn't make out the date numbers on this watch due to their being infinitesimally small, I almost had a serious mishap with a book deadline. Fortunately, the confusion was in my favor, but it caused a lot of undue stress in trying to meet a deadline that was off by a week. By then, I had just about had it with the thing.

I wanted a watch that I could see without having to hold it at just the right angle and I wanted a watch that I could glance at and determine what the date was without having to hold it up to my face as if I had macular degeneration. Or a giant blind spot. So, back to my original watch I went. If I got really concerned about it I could wear my plain, stainless steel watch. At that point, I didn't care about how toxic the battery was.

Getting faked out

A while back my husband and I stopped purchasing our favorite canned tomato products because of the issue with the BPA lining in cans. Finding an alternative lining for highly acidic foods, like tomatoes, is an issue for manufacturers and for the most part your choices are glass jars or the aseptic packages (those cardboard boxes that look like juice boxes). I could only find tomato paste in glass jars, so if I needed diced or whole canned tomatoes, I had to opt for the one product available in aseptic cardboard, which was Pomi. Pomi, unfortunately, wasn't certified organic, but it was an import from Italy where they use a lot fewer pesticides to begin with and their parent company was a certified producer of organic foods in Italy.[18] It was a trade-off for us as the Pomi products didn't taste as good as the organic brand we used to use and love, Muir Glen.

I had seen news reports saying that Muir Glen (a General Mills brand) was in the process of reformulating its cans and that, starting with the 2010 tomato crop, its tomato products would be canned without the use of BPA. This was great news, particularly in light of the fact that our annual pledge to u-pick tomatoes and can them ourselves in glass never seems to come to fruition here in Seattle where the tomato crop can be heinously paltry. Growing our own tomatoes for this purpose every year turns out to be an enormous lesson in frustration. The microclimate in our yard, just off Puget Sound, tends to remain cool for most of the day, even in the summer, and we are generally left with green tomatoes with just a few ripening each year.

However, in early December my husband popped into the grocery store on the way home from our annual family visit to see the Gingerbread Village at the Sheraton in downtown Seattle. Hank went in to pick up some items for making manicotti and, while he was reaching for the Pomi boxes, he noticed that the Muir Glen cans now advertised the fact that they were made with "enamel lined cans." He was excited when he got out to the car as he was thinking that these were the new BPA-free cans. He was so convinced about this labeling that he almost bought Muir Glen instead. But he knew better. I immediately went home to do some research and find out if, indeed, this was the case.

It wasn't. Those cans still had BPA in them and, as far as I was concerned, this was extremely misleading advertising on their part. Why mention the lining of your cans unless it was something significant? Most people don't care whether or not their cans are lined with white enamel. Many people, on the other hand, are concerned about whether or not their cans are lined with BPA. In looking around for current information on the cans, I saw that the Safe Mama website had followed up with Muir Glen about a month before this incident and had managed to nail down the gory details.

In summary, the fact was that they did not have BPA-free tomato products in cans yet on the shelves and that they wouldn't until sometime in 2011. Once they knew the date of production, the cans packaged after that production date could be considered BPA-free. Oddly enough, the customer service rep asked the writer from Safe Mama whether or not she would like the cans labeled as BPA-free.[19] Hopefully, with enough customer feedback, Muir Glen will know to label their cans with actual *useful* information. Until they start labeling the cans, it will still be a crapshoot distinguishing which cans have BPA and which don't. Even looking at the expiration date (a later date is more likely to indicate no BPA) doesn't guarantee anything.

Dirty money

Washington Toxics Coalition, in collaboration with Safer Chemicals, Healthy Families, released a report in early December 2010 explaining how their research showed that a considerable amount of BPA from thermal store receipts was ending up on paper money, most likely from people putting receipts in their wallets next to their bills. Ninety-five percent of the dollar bills they tested were positive for BPA, albeit in lower amounts than that found on the receipts. Because the BPA isn't chemically bound to the paper receipts (unlike in plastics), it comes off very easily, which is why the receipt issue is such a problem.

In tests mimicking the typical handling of receipts, about 2.5 micrograms of BPA was transferred from receipts to fingers in just 10 seconds. When the researchers rubbed the receipts, about 15 times as much BPA was transferred. While the high exposure to BPA (about 93% of Americans) was initially attributed to food consumption, it was starting to look like skin exposure was another, equally effective, route.[20] Between the handling of money and receipts, exposure to BPA through skin exposure was alarming to many people. What was next?

In reading these latest reports, I wasn't entirely concerned about my own personal risk from money because I never have cash on hand. We pretty much always use a credit card (for the free miles) that we pay off every month. My husband and I are notorious for never carrying money and we are always joking about living in a cash-free society because we hate dealing with cash. This bothers my mother to no end as she thinks having cash around is important in case of imminent societal collapse. Or, at the very least, a snowstorm, wherein a cascade of events will lead to the necessity of dollar bills. I don't mind having emergency money around, but I just won't use it on a daily, weekly or, really, monthly basis.

One thing this report did do was spark the idea in my mind that if I didn't think I would need the receipt for a purchase in the future I just wouldn't take it. It's not good for the cashier in either case, but they are already handling the receipt anyway. Since you really shouldn't be recycling BPA-laced receipts anyway (they contaminate the supply stream), I wasn't concerned about the fact that they were just throwing it out. It didn't have my signature or account information on it, so where it went wasn't an issue. After that, I started thinking more about my receipts and whether I needed them in the first place.

Unscented scent

My mom stopped by, as she does twice a week rain or shine, to drop off something or other, usually a newspaper clipping or something for the kids. I noticed immediately as she came into the house that, even though I know she doesn't wear perfume or use strongly scented soaps, there was an intense and strong scent that lingered for a long time even after she left. It took me a while to place what it was as it really had a chemical smell to it. I finally figured it out—it was probably some hand cream or lotion because it smelled a lot like those "unscented" lotions.

The issue with "unscented" lotions is that they aren't naturally unscented. Due to the chemicals and ingredients they are made out of, they have an inherently unpleasant odor to them which is then masked by a fragrance to make it not stink. In other words, the unscented product has artificial fragrance added to it to make it smell less like a vat of chemicals. As I became less and less exposed to scented products I became more and more sensitive to them, including the allegedly unscented ones. According to the FDA, even the label "fragrance-free" (which is different than the label "unscented") allows small amounts of fragrance to mask the fatty smell of the underlying product or any unpleasant odors. It's considered to be fragrance-free if there is no perceptible odor.

I considered asking my mom to stop wearing whatever it was that she had on, but I suspected that she probably wouldn't know what it was or wouldn't know what I was even smelling. The myriad makeup and body products and soaps she uses in the course of the day probably all had added fragrances in them. I would, more or less, be asking her to skip her entire toilette so that I wouldn't be exposed to the smell. The smell that she probably didn't even notice or would deny wearing since it wasn't a perfume or fragrance per se.

Non-toxic Christmas gifts

I figured that this year trying to find non-toxic Christmas gifts for the kids was going to be a huge struggle. But, as their requests came in and I looked a little closer into what they wanted, it ended up not being a big deal. Since Henry mostly wanted just Lego, which is probably the most inert toy you can buy (as far as chemicals go) since it's lead-free, PVC-free and BPA-free, his wishlist wasn't an issue. The cardboard box and little baggies that come with the sets were fine as well.

Emma wanted an array of stuffed animals, mostly sea creatures, with a horse thrown in for good measure. Books, clothing and natural candy canes rounded out the requests. Both kids also wanted gold leaf flakes to fill out their rock and gem collections, and this also wasn't an issue. It really was a non-toxic Christmas — at least from our end. The big problem would be controlling the other gifts that came in. Fortunately, that ended up being not a problem since they received more of the same type of gifts.

Henry wanted and asked my mom to get some Frango candies for Christmas. She buys these chocolate candies every year and he wanted some of the mint ones. The problem with Frangos is that they aren't organic, and I couldn't find the ingredient list for them ahead of time. I suspected artificial flavoring would be the biggest issue, but it was not really worth the fight since the impact would be minimal.

Trying to keep it all straight

I was four months into the project and still accidentally slipping up. Like eating some non-organic chips that I thought were organic and then realizing after the fact that the packaging had a non-stick Teflon-like coating inside. Or eating a slice of all-organic cake made by my husband but forgetting that he had baked it in the last non-stick item in the house (a Bundt pan which was later replaced). Or accidentally eating some leftover cheese for the kids that wasn't organic (they wouldn't eat the Organic Valley and pre-ferred only Tillamook). Then there was the absent-minded hand washing that went on in public restrooms because I wasn't paying attention and was pumping the soap out of habit, even when I was carrying my own soap.

Each time these slip-ups happened, particularly the ones that would affect my follow-up lab tests, I would be upset. I vowed to pay more attention to the soap issue but it was a real force of habit, kind of like retraining oneself to not grab paper towels in the bathroom and to use the blow dryers instead. It started to seem impossible to retrain myself on everything. Especially in the bathroom where I'm usually thinking about something else since my greatest mental breakthroughs occur during bathroom breaks. This, of course, got me thinking about the fact that it re-ally *shouldn't* take my full concentration day after day trying to avoid things that might poison me. It's really sad to think that, as Americans, we don't have the same protections from our products as Europeans do.

The European Union (EU) product safety laws follow the con-cept of the "precautionary principle" in that a manufacturer has to prove safety before an ingredient or chemical is allowed in a product. The opposite is true in the United States and Canada. Here one has to prove that an ingredient is deleterious or damag-ing before it can be removed and, even then, the FDA has no teeth to make a manufacturer recall a product. They can *recommend* that a product be recalled but you can pretty much guess where that goes. Of the tens of thousands of ingredients used in cosmetics alone, the EU has banned more than 1,000 chemical ingredients still in use by Americans today. In contrast, the U.S. has banned nine.[21]

This differentiation means that large companies have two different formulations for the same product — one for the EU and one for the U.S. The product sold in the EU must follow the precautionary principle and so the ingredients are considerably different from those in the product sold in the U.S. Why, one might ask, don't these companies, since they had to reformulate a "safe" version, just sell it in the U.S. and Canada as well?

It all comes down to culpability and lawsuits. If the manufacturer changes the formulation for the product sold in the United States they are opening themselves up to lawsuits because they are, essentially, admitting that their previous formulation might be dangerous. If people start coming forward with health claims after using a product for years they now have ammunition for their case. After all, why would the company change the formula if the previous one was safe? It's a catch-22 where American consumers are the losers.

Most people, and I used to be one of them, think that the FDA is protecting consumers. But the FDA neither tests the products that are on the market nor even requires manufacturers to supply safety information. They can't force a recall of a product and they really don't provide much in the way of protection in the first place. Yet, consumers still feel that if it is sold on the shelves, it must be safe. At the very least it must have been tested by someone. And usually, it has. Products get tested by the manufacturer and the FDA, in turn, relies on that data. But the companies are generally testing for an immediate physical reaction to a product or ingredient rather than long-term health consequences of daily exposure to small amounts of one of the thousands of chemicals that go into their products.

Figuring It All Out

Kissed by the sun

I had stopped getting my hair highlighted the previous Christmas so it had been about a year since I had it colored. The last time I went in I asked to have a lot of lowlights put in to match my natural coloring which is something close to a dark blonde. I had anticipated working on this book and suspected that hair coloring wasn't going to be in my future. While the darker hair dyes are the ones that have more suspicious toxins in them (69% of the dyes tested by the EWG may pose cancer risks[1]), ingredients in high-lighting and bleaching formulas are generally slightly better. The hazards also depend on what product you use. And, since 70% of American women color their hair, it seemed like a topic I shouldn't ignore just for the sake of reducing my exposure to toxins. Was there something out there that was effective, but relatively safe? I aimed to find out.[2] Plus, I was getting sick of my hair color and wanted it a little brighter looking.

The salon I had been going to, Habitude in Seattle, used an Aveda brand of hair coloring, Shades of Enlightenment™. Alleg-edly, 97% of the ingredients in this line were "naturally derived," meaning that they were made from plants and non-petroleum-based minerals. What I wanted to know was, what was in the re-maining 3%? The more gentle highlighting products on the market are ammonia-free and lack tar, lead, coal and other carcinogens. I decided to do some recon on the Aveda product and compare it with another line on the market, the blandly named Organic Color Systems. After my Brazilian Blowout experience, I didn't want another hair mishap. I emailed Aveda customer service to obtain a full ingredient listing for their product and, while I waited, I looked into Organic Color Systems.

According to their website, Organic Color Systems uses low levels of toxic pigments (aka PPD) to effectively color the hair. Their average level is 0.6%, as opposed to the legal maximum within the European Union which is 6%. But that was for *all* their hair color, not just for highlights. In addition, at least 89% of the Organic Color System line is naturally derived, with 10% made up of organically grown ingredients. I'm not sure if 10% warrants the "Organic" name, but whatever. Organic Color Systems products were allegedly free of ammonia, resorcinol, parabens and other toxic and carcinogenic ingredients commonly found in other products. This was helpful, but I wanted to know what was in the 11% not derived from natural ingredients. I emailed them as well for a full ingredient listing for a few of the colors in their natural range line of products.

Aveda got back to me the next day, offering up their full ingredient listing for their permanent hair-coloring formulas. The big red flags were the following, with the EWG hazard score in parentheses (1–10, with 10 being the most toxic):[3]

- Resorcinol (getting a whopping 10)
- p-Phenylenediamine (PPD — also ranking a 10)
- p-Aminophenol (ranking an 8–9)
- m-Aminophenol (ranking a 6)
- 1-Napthol (ranking a 6–8)
- Cocamidopropyl Betaine (ranking a 5)

I cringed at reading through the ingredient list because I knew resorcinol (a dihydroxy benzene) was a big bad boy in hair coloring and PPD was another issue. There was no way I could justify my way into using that product ever again.

Unfortunately, when I went to Whole Foods and looked at some of the alleged "herbal" highlighting products, even though they were ammonia- and resorcinol-free, the ones they carried (Naturtint and NaturColor) both had PPDs in them as well. So that left me with a choice. If I didn't want to expose myself to PPDs and still wanted to lighten my hair, I could go with some old-fashioned standbys. The most toxic option was using hydrogen peroxide (with a 3–6 ranking by EWG), but the results can be inconsistent and can result in orange hair, which isn't really something I was looking for.

The least toxic options were lemon juice, chamomile tea and honey. All three ingredients lighten hair to some degree. I decided to give that a whirl and see if I saw any lightening. Lemon juice, straight up, is inherently drying, so generally you add in some sort of natural oil to counteract it. In my case, I used jojoba oil in the mixture. Generally, when using lemon juice, you're supposed to sit

Non-toxic Home Hair Lightener

Ingredients

- ½ cup filtered water
- Chamomile tea, loose leaf (about 2 Tbsp)
- ½ tsp honey (optional—can make the hair very sticky)
- ½ cup fresh squeezed organic lemon juice
- 1 tsp jojoba oil (or other rich oils like olive oil or apricot oil)

Directions

Heat the water to almost a boil and add the chamomile tea. Steep for 15 minutes and strain, squeezing out the liquid. Add in the honey and stir to dissolve. When fully cool, add in the lemon juice and jojoba oil and stir to combine. Place in a spray bottle and shake before using. Spray onto damp hair. Sit in the sun (wearing non-toxic sunblock) until dry or use a hair dryer until dry. If your hair feels sticky, wash and let air-dry.

Note: I don't know how this will work on medium or very dark hair. My natural hair color is dark blond/light brown so it lightens up very quickly.

in the sun for the lightening to work. Since this was the middle of winter and, even if the sun decided to show itself, it wouldn't be very strong, I decided to go with the hair dryer and see if that worked. I guessed the active component was the heat, although I'm sure the UV exposure probably aided in the highlighting. In any case, I didn't have much choice in the matter.

Needless to say, the straight-up home hair lightener (*sans* the sun) didn't really do too much. So, I threw in some hydrogen peroxide to the mix (*à la* Sun-In) and tried it a few more times. I noticed some lightening going on and figured a few more applications would do the trick. However, as I was experimenting on my head I heard back from Organic Color Systems.

They emailed me the full listing of ingredients for their hair-lightening formula and I felt downright giddy reading through the listing. The only questionable ingredient was hydrogen peroxide. No ammonia or resorcinol. The pigments (or PPDs) were found in the formulas that laid down color, not removed it. A few weeks later I remembered a salon close to our house, Hazel Salon, used Organic Color Systems so I stopped my Sun-In home trial and booked an appointment.

Apple of my eye

It seemed ridiculous to be evangelically trying to remove toxins right and left in my food, drink, cleaners and personal care products and going to extremes to avoid the things I knew carried suspicious chemicals when I spent more than eight hours a day sitting underneath one of the most toxic items in the house. My laptop. If you had asked me months ago if there was such a thing as a non-toxic laptop, I would have looked at you funny because, really, it didn't seem possible. And it isn't. But there are some laptops on the market that are better than others, the best being the ones that don't have brominated flame retardants and aren't chock-full of PVCs and other contaminants.

While there are other options out there (including one made of bamboo), Apple's MacBook Pro claims to be the world's greenest laptop computer. Sure, it's "highly recyclable" and extremely energy efficient, but what does it have under the hood, chemically speaking? Apple products comply with the strict and bloatedly named European Directive on the Restriction of the Use of Certain Hazardous Substances in Electrical and Electronic Equipment, also known as the RoHS Directive. Chemicals restricted by the RoHS include lead, mercury, cadmium, chromium, brominated fire retardants and PBDEs. In addition, the MacBook Pro has an arsenic-free display glass, PVC-free internal cables, circuit board and power adapter cable and a PVC-free power cord. Finally, the MacBook Pro has a 10-hour battery charge. This is great because it means that I didn't have to sit with the laptop recharging on me (my old Windows laptop only held a charge for three hours, tops). This reduced my EMF exposure from charging all the time.[4]

Having a computer science degree and being a professional software developer, I was well aware of the almost religious following of Apple users versus Windows and, for that reason, I have always been turned off of Apple. Their followers can be over-the-top and, having spent 10 years developing software for Windows-based systems, I was much more comfortable "being a PC." But, given the stats on the Mac products, I was more than willing to switch over to the Mac side if only, at least, just to avoid toxins and have a battery that lasted more than three hours. I was in need of a new laptop anyway so this was a good investment for my work since I spend, generally, 10+ hours a day on my computer between writing and my "real" job.

One thing that I did have to avoid was getting a MacBook skin, which is a sticker that you can put on your laptop to dress it up. My husband has one on his laptop and I was looking into getting one that had sea life on it since my kids, my daughter especially, are into whales. It wasn't until I saw that the skins were made with vinyl that I looked into what kinds of plastics were used in the vinyl. Not too surprisingly, most if not all were made from PVC so I skipped the skin altogether. And, once more, I was amazed at how easy it was to overlook toxins in products.

Flooding with pineapples

A few weeks before Christmas, our area had a weather event that included a bit of warmth and a *lot* of rain. Usually the newscasters like to call it the cutesy Pineapple Express because this warm air and moisture generally originates from Hawaii or the South Pacific or somewhere tropical, fruity and delicious. Unfortunately for us, all that rain meant that our basement flooded a bit. I think, all told, I ended up wet-vacuuming up about 8 gallons of water, which is considerably less than three years ago when there was a good inch filling the entire basement. We clearly didn't have our water issues resolved yet, but it did bring into high relief for me some of the dangers of our flooring downstairs, as I spent every hour touching up the moisture building puddles.

Our basement is covered in a mix of slate tile, vinyl tiles, concrete and laminate. We had the carpeting pulled up in the family room and replaced with laminate five years earlier when we moved in because the carpet was disgusting. You could tell there was a decades-old mixture of water damage and cats involved down there. Given the fact that it is a partially underground basement in a very wet climate, replacing the carpet with more carpet sounded like a disaster in the making. And we didn't want to put down wood or bamboo because of the potential water issues. We were told not to remove the vinyl flooring that was under the carpet because of the very high probability that there was asbestos in the tile.

At the time, I didn't know anything about issues with plastic flooring so we opted for the wood knock-off laminate. After we got the floating tiles of laminate installed it stunk for a while, which isn't too surprising since most laminate has a resin in it made with formaldehyde and that off-gasses for a while. After five years, there isn't really anything off-gassing that I can tell or smell. However, there's still the old vinyl tile that covers the bedroom, hallways and large laundry and storage area down there. Since the vinyl tile is so old I don't know what other materials are in there, like PVC. Tearing up sample material for testing would be more hazardous than just leaving it alone.

The area that flooded this time around was by the bedroom door, hallway and the bathroom. The bathroom has stone tiles, but the hallway and bedroom do not, so that area was more of an issue. Particularly when I noticed that a chunk of vinyl tile had popped up when I was sucking up the water with the wet-vacuum. I can't really imagine anything bad coming of this particular loose tile exposure — it was soaking wet, after all — but it did remind me of all the potentially toxic asbestos-based flooring we had in the basement.

Our main floor is mostly hardwood flooring with tile in the main bathroom and some sort of linoleum in the kitchen and master bathroom. We do, unfortunately, have carpeting in the three bedrooms on the main floor. I wanted to get the carpeting removed in our bedrooms during this project because of the issue with synthetic carpets being treated with benzene and styrene and the fact that carpets trap toxins tracked in from outside and also hold a ton of dirt, mold and other spores.[5]

The issue with taking up the carpets led to the following problem. We had always assumed, since there are hardwoods in all the closets, that there was hardwood under the carpeting. But what condition was it in? What kind of refinishing would we need to have done to make it look decent? And what health effects can arise from refinishing hardwoods? It turned out that we just didn't have time to have the carpets pulled up during the project so it became a nonissue, but that didn't mean that I didn't look it up. I found one company in Seattle that claimed to do non-toxic floor finishing and "dustless" sanding. When we eventually did get the carpets removed and the floors finished, we were able to do it without dust or toxins.

On a final flooring note, our chicken coop has a removable linoleum piece over the chicken wire. The linoleum is there to keep their bedding from falling through the wire. The product we used, marmoleum, is a natural linoleum floor that is made with 100% natural ingredients such as linseed oil, cork, limestone, tree rosin and natural minerals. I've always been in love with marmoleum and, if we ever do any flooring replacement on the main floor (it wouldn't probably work very well in our wet basement), I would want to use marmoleum. As for the chickens, I didn't want them breathing in some off-gassing flooring and the natural linoleum has been working wonders at keeping things clean and secure.

Pine poisoning

At the end of the first week of Christmas break, I was blithely taking a shower. I heard my husband dutifully vacuuming the kitchen, which consistently gets coated by kid crumbs after every meal. I figured that breakfast must have resulted in a particularly high amount of cereal shedding and continued on without a thought. It wasn't until I stepped out of the bathroom that I was assaulted by the telltale fumes of a Pine-Sol invasion.

I don't know what possessed him to decide to clean the floors, let alone use Pine-Sol, but in any case the deed was done. I admit my reaction wasn't exactly very friendly but I was, quite frankly, irate. I'm sure he was expecting thanks rather than an attack, but I couldn't control my inner Non-Toxic Avenger. Lemon Fresh Pine-Sol is made out of thylene glycol butyl ether, which is on California's list of toxic air contaminants and it's easy to see why.[6] It contains neither pine nor lemon—nor anything resembling a forest. But it is breathtaking. People exposed to high levels of this chemical complain of nose and eye irritation (I'd add lung to that list) as well as headaches and vomiting.

So, I did what any unreasonable person would do. I opened up the windows in the affected areas and then holed up in Emma's bedroom with her, closed the door and opened her window until I could no longer smell the fumes or we left the house, whichever came first. I know my reaction to the situation was probably overly crazy but the last thing I needed was exposure to some more toxic fumes when I was just weeks away from my follow-up body burden testing. And, as such, I was being extra anal about avoiding toxins. This avoidance response would only get worse.

Numbness and pain: Part deux

The day after our basement flooded, I noticed the telltale symptoms of the numbness and tingling in my right hand again. In other words, the same symptoms I had experienced the previous August. Since it was just in my right hand I figured it had more to do with all the wet-vacc'ing I was doing, coupled with all the Christmas treats I was cooking for the kids' teachers. I initially ignored it but then it got progressively worse and I was feeling it predominately in my feet again. I tried ignoring it for a week and then I finally mentioned it to my husband. And that's when I started running back through my mental list of horrendous diseases that could be causing this. Clearly, at this point, it wasn't from a vitamin deficiency since I was still taking rather high levels of both Vitamin B12 and Vitamin D as supplements.

I immediately suspected it was something like multiple sclerosis (again) because of the episodic nature and the fact that I had felt mostly if not totally fine in the intervening three and a half months. By now it had been going strong for over two and a half weeks with no particular end in sight. I started researching again and, of course, numbness and tingling were some of the primary symptoms of MS. I then managed to comfort myself by thinking that, more reasonably, it was just me showing early signs of the disease my mom had just been diagnosed with since numbness and tingling in the extremities were also highly prevalent with that. We didn't have anyone in our family with MS, so I figured, following Occam's Razor (generally thought of as "the simplest explanation is more likely the correct one," but it's more complicated than that) that I was more likely to have the genetically predominant neuro-disease my mother had rather than something not in the family tree.

While I was going down this route, doing some research online and figuring that, if the symptoms were still there after the holidays I would finally go see a neurologist, I ran across an article about NutraSweet causing pain and numbness. While I hadn't been anywhere near NutraSweet in a very long time, I was struck by the fact that I had been drinking a protein beverage every day since the tingling had started. And I was drinking this same beverage back in August but not in between. I scoured through the ingredient listing, looking from something chemically obnoxious to hang my hat on, but no luck. The protein drink I had chosen was all-natural and I had picked it for that very reason.

It wasn't until I ran across a relatively uncommon side effect of the natural sweetener stevia that I put the two together. Stevia, which is a leaf herb, can cause numbness and muscle pain. Not only was I drinking a stevia-based protein drink, I had also picked up some stevia-sweetened soda for the holidays and had been drinking that over the last few weeks or so. Assuming that I was just barking up the wrong tree again, I didn't get my hopes up but, in any case, I decided to quite stevia cold turkey and see if the symptoms went away. I also stopped drinking all alcohol as that can aggravate peripheral neuropathy as well. Over the following week, the symptoms lessened each day until about one week after stopping the stevia, the only remaining symptom was the old threat of carpal tunnel in my right forearm.

It's entirely possible that the stevia had nothing to do with it and the numbness just went away and I'll experience it again sometime in the future, but it's also something I could easily test and challenge. However, having been scared twice in five months into thinking I had some incurable neurological disease certainly made me promise myself to stay as healthy as possible. With New Year's coming up I figured it was the perfect time to start planning on doing a three-week detox, starting on January 1 and ending with my follow-up body burden testing. I just needed to wade through the detox program set up for me months before by Dr. Hibbs and decide how I wanted to proceed.

Talking about the detox

I have to admit, the detox program that Dr. Hibbs had prescribed for me had me scared shitless. Which is one of the many reasons

I put if off until the end of the project. I really had made up some fabulous excuses about it, primarily not wanting to affect the lab results too much by doing something drastic, but, in reality, I was just stalling. The detox program they had suggested was based on some scientific studies of how to mobilize stored toxins in fat. It involved a pretty rigid program of diet, exercise, supplements and last, but definitely not least, sweating. Not just your ordinary, every-day sweating resulting from carrying up a laundry basket from the basement or some such thing, but four hours a day of sweating in a sauna. Sure, that time frame included breaks, but still — it was four hours a day. For four weeks. Because you are sweating for such long periods over such a long time, you need a lot of nutritional support and I was warned that most people felt like crap during the process. It was not really something I was eager to start up.

Furthermore, each week during the detox I would also meet with the doctor at least twice to check in and make sure I was do-ing okay. This involved not just talking and taking vital signs, but also doing blood work if things weren't looking good. Each day of the detox would involve at least 30 minutes of exercise followed by 4 hours of sweating (assisted by hefty dosages of niacin) and a fairly restricted diet of organic fruits and vegetables, protein, fat and carbohydrates, all measured out to make sure I was getting the correct balance. In addition, there were numerous supplement and nutritional support aids to be bought and consumed to make sure I didn't crump, which was the term my mom used to use as a hos-pice nurse when her patient was about to permanently keel over.

In light of the fact that my initial heavy metal lab results weren't dramatically high, my levels of DDE were low and the PCBs were undetectable, I was less excited about going through a month of hell to achieve something probably not too effective on numbers that were more or less nonexistent. In other words, most of the toxins that were found in my body were of the sort that were processed fairly quickly out of the body — the high parabens, phthalates and volatile solvents levels were also contaminants that were direct-exposure related and I was fairly confident that sweat therapy detox wasn't going to have a tremendous effect on the final results. Finally, my other big justification for switching up the detox was because of the readers of this book.

I was concerned about making the things I did during this project mostly accessible to readers. So, for those following along at home, I wanted it to be at least somewhat reasonable that similar changes could be made by them as well. A four-week sweatfest, which, when you add up the supplement costs and the sauna fees, ends up being quite expensive in addition to being time-consuming. And you need physician support to do it safely. All in all, it would be a huge turnoff for most people. It certainly was for me and I was willing to subject myself to a lot of things.

For months I had been trying to figure out what to do about the detox. Since I had punted it to the end of the project it was like there was a giant, sweaty gorilla waiting for me at the end of the tunnel. I finally decided to take elements of the detox program and make it more doable not just for me, but for readers as well. I decided to follow the exercise and dietary restrictions as recommended—adding in additional supplements as well—and to do a daily lymphatic dry-brushing as recommended. I threw in some short home-style baths and other treatments to round it out. The latter included Epsom salt baths (for sweating and because Epsom salts are purported to help draw toxins out of the skin), bentonite clay baths (for the same purposes) and weekly massages. Massage helps move toxins out of the body and the place where I got my massages, Ballard Health Center, also had a hot tub where I could sweat it out for 20 minutes before my weekly appointments.

As for the exercise, I worked out daily for at least 30 minutes, mostly walking or dancing. The lymphatic dry-brushing actually felt great. Before I took my daily shower, I used a bristle brush and swept it up and down my skin (always in the direction toward my heart) to help move lymph around and help detox. Or some such thing. I'm fairly skeptical about pretty much anything that doesn't have some scientific studies behind it, but I was willing to fly with some of these things (like the Epsom salts and bentonite clay) for the purposes of this book. As long as there was some potential detox action associated with it. Plus, they didn't exactly hurt and may even have helped.

The diet consisted of mostly organic fruits and vegetables (60%–70% of my intake) with some salmon, organic chicken and eggs. I limited the dairy—no butter and no milk or cheese (taking calcium and Vitamin D supplements, of course). I eliminated all processed flours and wheat. For grains I stuck to whole oats, brown rice and quinoa. I also ate a lot of beans and corn. Since the original detox plan recommended also eating a tablespoon of olive oil (or similar oils) a day to help get rid of the toxins that are mobilized, I added in a lot of fats that way. I also ate a lot of olives and nuts to round things out. While I didn't feel hungry or deprived much, I did lose weight, mostly because all those fruits and vegetables are filling, as are lean meats and beans. I did occasionally splurge with some dark chocolate, but as I went through the detox, I wasn't as interested in it. I also eliminated all coffee (regular and decaf) and drank a lot of Yogi Detox Tea, which was actually tasty and has herbs in it that allegedly help detox your liver. I completely eliminated alcohol as well and relied mainly on purified water for hydration.

As for the supplements, I took my usual daily multivitamin, calcium, turmeric, B12, D3, C and added in additional Vitamin C and flax seed oil. I tried taking chlorella the first two days of the detox although I was wary of it. Again, it's supposed to help with detoxing the body. My mom gave me some Sun Chlorella tablets but she warned me that she had some serious stomach problems with them. After reading about chlorella online, I saw that many people had issues with vomiting when taking it. I started out at a really low level and felt okay on the first day. The second day I doubled the dose and had a phenomenal headache, almost like a migraine. I didn't know whether or not it was linked with the chlorella, but I never get headaches and I only rarely get migraines. But my migraines are pretty easy to identify and this was definitely not a migraine. It was some weird, induced headache. Some might argue it was from going through detox, but I won't know because I never took any more chlorella to test that theory.

In addition to all this, I made sure that I got at least 7 hours of sleep at night, stretched twice a day and meditated for 30 minutes a day. This last thing I did not just for relaxation purposes but also because it's been shown to reduce cholesterol, blood pressure and blood sugars. At least, that's what Dr. Oz claims. Finally, I also decided, since I wasn't doing the full-on sweat therapy, to do a once-a-week juice fast. Fasting is supposed to help rid the body of toxins and juice fasting is easier on the system than water fasting. I figured a weekly rest for my digestive tract might be in order. It didn't last long. I really only made it through the first week and just never had the time to do it again since it required a bit of planning.

Whether or not any of the things I did for those four weeks really helped squeeze any additional toxins out of me will never be known but I felt great. I got a lot of exercise; ate super-clean with a lot of high-fiber, high-nutrient foods; got pampered in the bath and the sauna, and with massage; and between all that and meditation, I was *über*-relaxed. The truth would reveal itself in the follow-up testing results. Scheduling the follow-up body burden labs was a breeze in comparison to getting them rolling the first time around. I went in and had them done, forked over the entire contents of my wallet and then some and waited for the results.

The high cost of organics

Before the detox, my husband and I usually bought a considerable amount of organic foods in our weekly shopping so I was really quite surprised by how expensive it was when we switched to 100% organic everything. Of course, I could have gotten around some of that by choosing items that were sustainably grown and not certified organic, but I wanted to be sure I didn't have any exposure to pesticides. It ended up being more costly than our usual shopping and definitely way more expensive than buying conventional.

However, I would argue that the costs are worth it in terms of soil preservation (buying organic means that better farming practices were employed) and long-term health costs. For starters, it's hard to find much in the way of organic junk food, although I suppose it can be done. The reduction in hormones, antibiotics and pesticides going into my food and, therefore, me just means I'm that much healthier and won't have long-term health effects from consistently eating conventionally grown, produced and manufactured foods. It was worth it in other regards, too; mostly in relation to flavor, quality and safety.

Eating out was definitely a gigantic pain. Most coffee shops didn't have organic milk even if they had organic coffee. Finding an organic restaurant just meant that we were extremely limited. And that was here in Seattle. I would imagine that in the rest of the U.S. options are downright bleak. But I always asked for organic options and I hoped that, by doing so, the message would get picked up and the restaurants would start offering more organic choices.

Consuming foods contaminated by pesticides and herbicides, combined with the increased risk of foodborne illnesses (like *E. coli* outbreaks), all add up from a health and human services' perspective. Health care costs, as well as quality of life, are heavily impacted by disease and, while you may not be paying for it up front, you are paying for it down the road in terms of environmental exposure, illness and disease, sometimes terminal.

A higher cost of living seems to be the price to pay for a non-toxic lifestyle in general. Most consumable products (like personal care products and household cleaners) themselves are cheaper because they are simple and can oftentimes be homemade, but replacing a lot of what you have already, especially durable goods (like pots and pans and clothing, for example), for non-toxic versions can be expensive. Replacing items when they are gone or worn out with non-toxic alternatives would help allay the costs since the alternatives are no more or less expensive in many cases (except food). But, again, lowering the risks to your health and your children's health is worth the cost, even if it's incremental. And, for truly suspicious products, allocating money for their early replacement is worth it in the long run.

The moment of truth: XRF analyzer

When it came time to test some of our household products for heavy metals, Erika Schreder at Washington Toxics Coalition helped me out yet again. She was the one who initially counseled me about where to find body burden testing and which tests would be accessible to me. This time around she saved my skin by offering up the use of the Coalition's XRF analyzer gun. Because these machines are expensive (generally around $30,000), buying one wasn't exactly practical and renting one was costly. And also, I wanted to make sure I was using an XRF analyzer that would give a scientifically significant analysis. Cheaper ones exist on the market, but the results wouldn't have been as definitive. In any case, in early February we managed to find a time that worked for both of us and I trooped down to their offices with a large bag of common household items to test out.

X-ray fluorescence (XRF) analyzers are widely used by government regulators and product manufacturers to test for hazardous materials in consumer products without destroying the sample being analyzed. They can test for chemical elements like chlorine, lead, cadmium, arsenic, mercury, tin and antimony. They can also tell you if a product is made out of PVC, which came in handy with the stuff I brought in.

After scaring me with some results they had just gotten regarding the amount of formaldehyde in crib sheets, infant clothes and pretty much all textiles that aren't organic, we got down to business. Erika had her intern, Rachel, join us to show her how to use the analyzer which meant that I got to learn alongside as well. After Erika explained the safety hazards of shooting x-rays at people and calibrated the gun, we were ready to begin.

Rachel had brought with her two sets of Lego toys — one from 1979 and one from 1984. The significance of this was that Lego changed the materials of their plastic toys between these dates. Modern-day Lego toys are generally fine, although the clear plastic pieces are made from polycarbonate and, most likely, contain BPA. So, it is essential that I make sure the kids aren't sucking on those particular pieces.

In the 1979 set, the red Lego brick measured at over 7,000 ppm (parts per million) cadmium. In contrast, the 1984 red (and yellow) bricks found no cadmium detected. Cadmium, which is a known carcinogen, can hinder brain development, similar to lead. Even though our kids play with recently manufactured Lego, I mention this because we have been offered sets of Lego from yesteryear that somebody or other's grandparent had been storing in their basement. Usually we refuse them because of the mildew and high ick factor of these long-lost treasures, but now there's more reason to be concerned about plastic toys made in the 1970s. What's the significance of 7,000 ppm cadmium? While there are no federal limits of cadmium in children's toys (yet), 7,000 ppm is extremely high. For comparison, the European toy standard is 75 ppm.[7] In other words, really, anything about 100 ppm is high — 7,000 ppm is insanely high.

Also scoring high in cadmium was the charm on a bracelet given to Emma for Christmas. The bracelet itself was okay, not registering lead or cadmium, but the holly charm tested in at 1,440 ppm cadmium and 320 ppm lead. The federal limit for lead is 300 ppm. I took off the charm and gave her back the bracelet. I shuddered to think of how many times I had caught Emma with that bracelet covered in slobber. She has a bad habit of sucking on her metal bracelets and I really didn't want that charm going back in her mouth. We tested another one of Emma's bracelets, but this one came out clean — no cadmium even on the peace sign charm. It was just made out of a titanium zinc alloy which was a relief as I didn't want to have to throw out all her toys that I had brought.

I also brought in one of my necklaces that I used to wear quite frequently but had stopped wearing at the beginning of the project. It was mostly made out of metal, but I wasn't sure what kind. Since it was inexpensive jewelry I figured it contained something suspicious. XRF analysis confirmed I was right in a big way. It tested in at just under 1,500 ppm lead, which is way above the federal limit. What was more amazing to me was, at the time of the testing, certain lawmakers were trying to rollback recent legislation requiring product manufacturer testing of kids' toys and jewelry for heavy metals. Testing of children's jewelry was clearly not happening prior to this legislation and look what was out on the market because no one was doing it! Furthermore, what about all the *adult* products on the market that should also be tested? How many adults are walking around wearing a lead bomb around their necks? That necklace sat directly on my skin and, with the rain, sweating and regular wear and tear, who knows what impact, if any, there was?

Next up were the plastics. I brought in a squeezy "rubber" bath toy shaped like a fish that squirted water. It tested as PVC with greater then 25% chlorine. The blue dinosaur bath toy was PVC. The plastic snake was PVC. The squeaky Jesus Christ lizard (aka Green Basilisk lizard) tested in at 16% chlorine on his belly and 17% chlorine on his neck flap. Henry's watchband was PVC with a little chromium thrown in for good measure, but the watch itself was okay. In addition to the chlorine, all these PVC products most likely contain phthalates as well. And they get sucked on, chewed on and who knows what else.

My watchband, the one that I went back to after sweating it out with the Sprout steamy undecipherable watch, came back testing out okay. The watchband on my Timex sports watch wasn't PVC. There was 18 ppm bromine found, but the amount was so small it wasn't significant (anything over 1,000 ppm bromine is considered high). The watch itself was okay. So, I happily put my watch back on and considered how much energy and thought went into trying to find out whether or not this particular consumer product was "safe," which is something I shouldn't have to do myself.

We had a set of china from Korea that my uncle bought for my mom as a gift when he served there in the military (ca. 1960s). I brought in a plate and it tested in at 8,300 ppm lead. Lead glazing and the detailing on the china was probably what was giving such high readings but Erika suggested that there weren't too many conclusive studies showing a problem with eating off lead plates, although these tested particularly high. In any case, I certainly wasn't going to use them again.

Last, but not least, were the chargers for my two laptops. The first one we tested was for my old Dell laptop. The cord tested as PVC with 1.3% antimony. The charger itself contained 1,390 ppm bromine and 1,800 ppm antimony (a catalyst with flame retardants). It's quite common for electronics to contain brominated flame retardants because they get hot when they're charging. Again, anything above 1,000 ppm bromine is considered high. In contrast, the laptop charger for my new Mac contained... Nothing detectable. It's always a great feeling to have something confirmed because you can't tell by just looking at a product if it contains something that is potentially a problem.

The only other thing I brought in for testing that didn't register anything potentially hazardous was Henry's rain boots. I thought for sure they were made out of PVC with some lead in the paint on them, but they were fine. Erika couldn't find anything in them in spite of testing different sections. Besides those and my watch, everything else that I brought in had something suspicious and over the limits. To be fair, I didn't exactly bring in completely inert items. I brought things I had concerns about. But that just left me wondering what else (toys, costume jewelry) had problems and what was okay. Again, I couldn't tell just by looking at things. And I certainly couldn't rely on any consumer standards protecting us either.

Lab results reckoning

It was tough waiting for the follow-up body burden lab results to come in. Since it takes weeks to get the results I had to stop myself from bugging Dr. Hibbs every few days to see if he'd seen anything. The first lab result I got back was for the heavy metal whole blood. It was just a teaser for things to come. After tracking down all the lab results for me, Bastyr sent me the rest of the results in one fell swoop. To make things easier, here they all are, side by side, before and after.

Table 2.

Toxic Element (in whole blood)*	Before (µg/L)	After (µg/L)	Reference Range
Arsenic	4.4	4.9	<9.0
Cadmium	0.7	0.7	<2.0
Cobalt	0.2	0.3	<1.5
Lead	0.7	0.7	<3.0
Mercury	1.0	< 0.6	<5.0
Toxic Elements (in urine)	**Before (µg/g creatinine)**	**After (µg/g creatinine)**	**Reference Range**
Aluminum	1.9	Not detected	<35
Arsenic	21	9	<117
Barium	1.4	0.7	<7
Cadmium	0.6	0.3	<1
Cesium	4.2	5.3	<10
Lead	0.4	0.3	<2
Mercury	1.3	0.6	<4
Nickel	4.5	3.2	<12
Thallium	0.1	0.3	<0.5
Tin	0.1	0.2	<10
Tungsten	0.9	0.2	<0.4
Volatile Solvents (whole blood)	**Before (ppb)**	**After (ppb)**	**95th Percentile (ppb)**
Benzene	Not detected	Not detected	0.26
Ethylbenzene	0.1–0.3	0.1–0.3	0.11
Styrene	Not detected	Not detected	0.12
Toluene	Not detected	Not detected	0.68
m,p-Xylene	0.4–1.3	0.4–1.3	0.34

o-Xylene	Not detected	Not detected	0.09
Hexane	140.02	176.96	≤200
2-Methylpentane	47.1	55.6	≤84
3-Methylpentane	38.7	105.7	≤128
Isooctane	4.06	8.97	≤30.60
Chlorinated Pesticides (serum)	**Before (ppb)**	**After (ppb)**	**95th Percentile (ppb)**
DDE	0.36	0.41	12.10
DDE (lipid adjusted)	71.9 ng/g lipid	96 ng/g lipid	1860 ng/g lipid
DDT	Not detected	Not detected	0.13
Dieldrin	Not detected	Not detected	0.14
Heptachlor epoxide	Not detected	Not detected	0.13
Hexachlorobenzene (HCB)	Not detected	Not detected	0.19
Mirex	Not detected	Not detected	0.09
Oxychlordane	Not detected	Not detected	0.27
Trans-Nonachlor	Not detected	Not detected	0.47
Cholesterol	170 mg/dl	146 mg/dl	≤ 200 mg/dl
Triglycerides	122 mg/dl	87 mg/dl	35–160 mg/dl
Total lipids	5 g/L	4 g/L	
Polychlorinated Biphenyls (PCBs) (serum)	**Before (ppb)**	**After (ppb)**	
Dioxin-like PCBs: PCB 118, PCB 126, PCB 156, PCB169	Not detected	Not detected	
Nondioxin-like PCBs: PCB 74, PCB 138, PCB 153, PCB 180	Not detected	Not detected	

Phthalates	Before (ug/g creatinine)	After (ug/g creatinine)	95% Reference Interval
MEHHP	255	254	≤1,253
MEHP	36	18	≤209
MEOHP	74	58	≤569
MEtP	>2500	539	≤3,143
Parabens	Before (ug/g creatinine)	After (ug/g creatinine)	95% Reference Interval
Butylparaben	3	6	≤36
Ethylparaben	78	8	≤282
Methylparaben	>2500	25	≤2,995
Propylparaben	>2500	8	≤959

* Note: Lithium levels went up into the normal range and molybdenum levels went back down into normal range.

I'd like to think that I have some great explanations for why a few things went up after this project. Some weren't statistically significant so it's not worth mentioning them directly, but the increased readings (for the DDE and some of the volatile solvents like hexane and the methylpentanes) are most likely due to the fact that my detox mobilized more of them out of storage and into my bloodstream for removal. Doing fat biopsies, again, would have been more conclusive and the interpretation of the results seen here can only be guesswork without further, long-term follow-up testing.

As for the heavy metals, arsenic went up slightly in my blood, but down considerably in my urine. Both blood and urine showed a marked decrease in mercury and there was a slight drop in lead in my urine. Across the board there was a decrease in most toxic elements. The rest of the volatile solvents remained the same or undetected. The PCBs remained undetectable as did almost all of the chlorinated pesticides (except DDE, a metabolite of DDT, mentioned above).

The most notable drop was in a couple of the phthalates and all but one of the parabens. MEHHP must be a bugbear to get rid of because that didn't drop at all. I couldn't find much information on that particular phthalate, so I don't know what significance it has. The rest of the phthalates fell by almost half or more. The parabens were another story. Except for the butylparaben (which was low to begin with), they literally fell off the map. I must have been literally drinking methylparaben and propylparaben before or something.

I'll be the first to admit that four or so months doesn't give one's body a whole lot of time to recover from exposures to a variety of potentially hazardous chemicals so I was happy to see a decrease in several things in spite of this. What it tells me is that even a short-term reduction in exposures can have a profound effect on what is circulating through your system. Lifestyles changes and chemical avoidance, over years, can be significant when it comes to health and disease.

Finally, what I found particularly interesting was the large drop in my cholesterol and triglycerides. My cholesterol went from 170 just four months earlier to 146 and my triglycerides went from 122 to 87. Triglycerides are a type of fat that gets stored if you eat too many calories. All I can say about the drop there is that I was probably depleting my fat stores during detox. I lost about six pounds overall so it makes sense that there was a decrease. I'm astounded at how many points my cholesterol dropped. It hasn't been this low since I enrolled in a psychology experiment at the UW during my freshman year in college where they took my cholesterol reading and told me it was (falsely) high to see my reaction. That 145 reading back in 1989 was nowhere near the 210 they told me it was. And, now, 20 years later, it's right back down there. You can't tell me that eating tons of homegrown eggs gives you high cholesterol.

Final health updates

In January, Hank was severely neutropenic due to the chemo that he takes to keep his cancer from multiplying and that will hopefully push him into complete remission one day. What this means was that he pretty much didn't have any white blood cells. Since he rides the bus to work with all manner of sick people, I made him either drive or work from home until he got a GCSF shot to help restore his white blood cells. Or, more accurately, to help regulate the production of neutrophils within his bone marrow. Hank's oncologist also had to reduce his chemo dosage because of the neutropenia.

In spite of the chemo reduction, he continued doing well. They further reduced his steroid immune suppressants such that by the time I submitted this manuscript he was off it completely. His liver function continued to do well, and he showed only small signs of graft versus host attacking his skin. Even his oncologist—the same oncologist who had given him a probabilistic three-year death sentence exactly three years earlier—was surprised at how well he was doing.

While he certainly didn't go into complete remission during the course of the project, he did end up getting off some of the nastier drugs he was on. Whether or not his cancer levels and his body's ability to handle his cancer and medications better had something to do with less inundation by other toxins is not something I can speculate on. I'd like to think it helped, but I honestly don't care what the cause was. The result was that he was better and that was all I wanted.

My son, Henry, was faring about the same at the end of the project as he was at the beginning. Since he already ate a pretty Feingold-esque diet (minimal colorants, additives, etc.) I didn't expect to see much neurological improvement due to decreased toxin exposure. His behavioral and social issues continued, some getting better and some getting worse over the course of the school year. During his third grade school year his teacher did report a dramatic drop in disruptions as compared to previous years, yet his impulsive outbursts still occurred occasionally.

The damage that was potentially done to him from toxins early on was, well, already irreversibly done and it would take time and maturity and services and medication to help him overcome all those things the rest of us take for granted. My hope for him is that he outgrows many of his issues just as other family members and I have. The tics, the anxiety, the OCD—all those things can be managed later in life or outgrown. Learning social skills will always be a challenge, but he brings so much to those who truly know him that I have no doubt that he will one day be happy, successful and less anxious. It's getting there that's the struggle.

As for me, I never did have a recurrence of the numbness, tingling and pain that I associated with the stevia. Until I test it again I won't know for sure, but all I *can* claim is that, during the entire length of the project I didn't have any more migraines and I didn't get sick more than once in spite of the fact that my daughter brought home back-to-back colds during that entire time—and I usually get one cold a month from her during most years. My immune system must have been a lot stronger to have fended off her usual viral brigade.

I hope that by bringing to light the potential health effects of so many of the chemicals and neurotoxins that our bodies, our babies and our children get exposed to will stem the tide of autism and the myriad cancers and diseases that plague modern Americans. I sincerely disagree with the slogan "better living through chemistry" when it causes such a decrease in quality of life for so many at the same time.

Wrapping It Up

It was the best of times

It's been a few months since I had my final body burden labs done and the pressure to stick to non-toxic avenging is off. In other words, I could potentially go back to a toxic product free-for-all and do whatever the hell I wanted. I could slather myself with whatever creams and cosmetics I wanted and stuff my face with processed, high-fructose corn syrup and pesticide-laden products wrapped in nonstick packaging. But I can't. I can't go back. Living with these changes for almost five months made them habits, made me used to the new products and made me want to continue. Everything.

The only thing that has slipped is trying to stick to 100% organic food all the time. Which isn't to say that I'm not trying. I still buy all organic when I go to the grocery store, but I'm not as nutty about it when we go out to eat. Although, I will still only buy organic wine since I continue to be haunted by those "pesticides in wine" studies.

But I cannot deny that some changes were easier and/or better than others. And some were just downright fun. And I thought it would make sense to do a short rundown of which changes I did and didn't like and what changes, if any, I've made since then.

Hands down, my favorite changes thanks to the project were:

Getting plants for air filtering: I love growing food plants out in the yard (all organic, of course), but I didn't think that I'd enjoy having house plants so much. They have added such a nice, tropical feel to the house I ended up buying even more after the project ended. I just needed to sneak them in one at a time since Henry was still complaining about them.

New vacuum cleaner: I really don't have much to say besides the fact that I love it. It doesn't stink and I know it's doing a bang-up job of cleaning the house. I may not necessarily be vacuuming as often, but the house stays a lot cleaner now with the HEPA filter.

Getting rid of Teflon in the kitchen: We really don't need any nonstick pots or pans in the kitchen. Nobody does. There are so many other options out there that are inexpensive, easy to care for and last a long time that there's no excuse for chunks of Teflon in your food.

Eating all organic: While it's definitely more expensive, it's also definitely worth avoiding the pesticides and other chemical residue on what I eat. If we are eating out, we try to find a place with organic or sustainable options but if there aren't any, I don't sweat it.

Using 100% clean body products: I take great pleasure in knowing that absolutely everything I put on my body is about as non-toxic as you can get without them being edible. From my hair to my makeup, skincare, soap, deodorant and toothpaste, I know nothing is poisoning me via the largest organ in my body.

Detoxing and exercise: While the detox seemed long, I got a lot out of it and have been keeping up with an occasional Epsom bath as well as bimonthly deep-tissue massages (with the hot tub!). As for the exercise, it's become a habit that I have continued along with the stretching. Dry-brushing feels great so that is something I still do, plus I like the way my skin feels. I've updated my diet to include a lot more vegetables, limited my sugar and flour intake and continued with fruits and lean meats—all of it being organic, of course.

It was the worst of times

Not everything was a party (clearly) and there were some things I definitely struggled with. However, in spite of some problems, I'm still doing pretty much everything that I did during the project. Nothing was so difficult that I reverted back to a more hazardous product or method of living. Okay, maybe a few slipped back in there.

Deodorant: Once I found the right combination of ingredients to avoid the irritated brown skin problem, life in Pittsville was good. Scooping out homemade deodorant sometimes is a little more of a pain than I feel like doing when I'm running late in the morning, so some days I just use the unscented Ban Roll-On. I generally use either Ban or homemade deodorant depending on the day and how much sweating I'll be doing. But I haven't gone back to a scented, more toxic product.

Mascara and eyeliner: I have to say, the alternatives I've been using just don't work as well as the commercial products. The eyeliner doesn't provide the same sort of coverage and the mascara smudges like nobody's business. If I'm having a sneezing fit (which is often), the mascara will smear all over the place. I will continue to look for a better substitute or just not wear any.

Hair color: I found that the natural homemade lighteners just didn't do anything without the sun, including my homemade version of Sun-In. I continued using the Organics Hair Color System at Hazel Salon because, although it has a few sketchy glycols in it, overall it's the best out there.

Laundry detergent: While I love our BioKleen laundry detergent, the stink eventually builds up in our clothes and renders them unwearable. Particularly those clothes that see a lot of sweat (hello, homemade deodorant!) or ones that get worn several times or are dirty. As a remedy, I now occasionally will wash our clothes in petroleum-based laundry detergent to get them freshened up, but I try to choose an unscented "safe for baby" version. And sometimes you just have to call in the big guns and use something like

Tide. Sigh. But then we switch back to BioKleen and are good for a while.

Mold cleaning: Our shower stall was just as stubborn as could be and, while I didn't go back to using X-14 for cleaning it, I now use an occasional mix of water with a little bleach to get the more pesky areas. The bleach stinks but it's not as eye burning and lung searing as the X-14. I try to use it as infrequently as possible and will continue to look for a more earth- and lung-friendly alternative.

What does it all even mean?

So, where does all this leave us? It's still an uphill, daily battle trying to determine whether or not a product I pick up at the store will poison me. Only the over-educated consumers have enough ammo to arm themselves against the onslaught of chemicals that exist, even in products that claim they are natural, organic or unscented as shown by my lab tests. Just getting rid of your Teflon pans doesn't mean you aren't exposed to Teflon-like coatings at every turn in your kitchen and on your clothes and in your dental floss. Eating organic will prevent exposure to all manner of pesticides, but how many Americans are willing, or can afford, to spend the extra money to ensure that their family is eating cleaner, less risky food?

And even if an individual wanted to find out what kind of toxic body burden they have, it's unlikely they'll ever know. Access to the few laboratories that run most of these tests can be difficult, or even impossible, unless the people wanting to be tested are part of a research study. On top of the issue of inaccessibility is affordability. Not every curious person is willing to shell out thousands of dollars for testing and, since these tests can't be considered diagnostic without cause, it's unlikely that health insurance would ever cover them. In some regards I'm lucky because I know what toxins are in my body. I also know what I can do to prevent more from coming in and what I can do to get out more of what's left. But that's not the case for the vast majority of citizens.

Individual choices can make a difference, but what Americans need is an overhaul of the Toxic Substances Control Act. We need a replacement that is more in alignment with the EU's precautionary principle standard. We need one that protects consumers rather than leaving them at risk of potentially applying tens, if not hundreds, of suspicious products and chemicals every day. How long do we have to wait for our government representatives to get the message that we deserve better? That they and their families deserve better, even if it's at a cost to their corporate constituents? Because, in the end, those same corporations will have to help foot the bill of the healthcare costs associated with long-term usage of hazardous chemicals by way of cancer, asthma and who knows what else lurking on the horizon?

I hope that by the time this book is in print and on the bookshelves and in your hands that the Safe Chemicals Act will have replaced the Toxic Substances Control Act and that the Safe Cosmetics Act will have also passed as well. These two updates to our failing safety system certainly do not solve many of the problems, but it's a start.

Finally, please support organizations such as Commonweal, Washington Toxics Coalition, Toxipedia and Environmental Working Group that give consumers the knowledge to make better choices. If you have been concerned about what you've read here, let your legislators know. About the toxic chemicals that is. Not about my mental wellbeing.

Notes

Part 1: Laying It All Out

1. "Toxic Chemicals in Washington Residents—Pollution In People." pollutioninpeople.org (accessed September 30, 2010).
2. "Overview Clinical Laboratory Improvement Amendments (CLIA)." Centers for Medicare & Medicaid Services. cms.gov/clia/ (accessed February 22, 2011).

Part 2: Getting Started

1. "Viewing Poisons at Our National Parks." Miller-McCune. miller-mccune.com/environment/viewing-poisons-at-our-national-parks-20350/ (accessed September 30, 2010).
2. "XRF Analyzer Testing Toys For Lead." Atlas Inspection Technologies. atlas-inspection.com/xrf-lead-testing.html (accessed October 22, 2010).
3. "Polycarbonate." Wikipedia, the free encyclopedia. en.wikipedia.org/wiki/Polycarbonate (accessed September 2, 2010).
4. Morgan, Erinn and Gina White. "Eyeglass Frame Materials." All About Vision. allaboutvision.com/eyeglasses/eyeglass_frame_materials.htm (accessed August 20, 2010).
5. "Glass Nose Pads." Nose Pad King Home Page. stores.nosepadking.com/-strse-Glass-Nose-Pads/Categories.bok (accessed August 20, 2010).
6. "PVC Guide." Center for Health, Environment & Justice. chej.org/campaigns/pvc/ (accessed August 15, 2010).
7. "CDC—Lice—Head Lice." Centers for Disease Control and Prevention. cdc.gov/parasites/lice/head/index.html (accessed October 2, 2010).
8. "CDC—Lice—Head Lice—Treatment." Centers for Disease Control and Prevention. cdc.gov/parasites/lice/head/treatment.html (accessed October 2, 2010).

9. "ACF Newsource — Toxic Shampoo." ACF Newsource.org. acfnewsource
   .org/environment/toxic_shampoo.html (accessed October 2, 2010).

10. "PANNA: Lindane Action Plan Must Include U.S. Ban." Pesticide Ac-
    tion Network. panna.org/legacy/panups/panup_20051019.dv.html (ac-
    cessed October 5, 2010).

11. Fitzgerald, Randall. *The Hundred-Year Lie: How to Protect Yourself from
    the Chemicals That Are Destroying Your Health.* New York: Plume, 2007.

12. Lau, Karen, W. Graham McLean, Dominic Williams, and C. Vyvyan
    Howard. "Synergistic Interactions between Commonly Used Food Ad-
    ditives in a Developmental Neurotoxicity Test." Oxford Journals | Life
    Sciences & Medicine | Toxicological Sciences. toxsci.oxfordjournals.org
    /content/90/1/178.abstract (accessed April 13, 2011).

13. Fitzgerald, Randall. *The Hundred-Year Lie: How to Protect Yourself from
    the Chemicals That Are Destroying Your Health.* New York: Plume, 2007.

14. "Phthalate." Wikipedia. en.wikipedia.org/wiki/Phthalate (accessed
    September 15, 2010).

15. Fitzgerald, Randall. *The Hundred-Year Lie: How to Protect Yourself from
    the Chemicals That Are Destroying Your Health.* New York: Plume, 2007.

16. Fitzgerald, Randall. *The Hundred-Year Lie: How to Protect Yourself from
    the Chemicals That Are Destroying Your Health.* New York: Plume, 2007.

17. Rung International. "Allura Red Ac." Food colours, food products, food
    additives. foodcolourworld.com/products/allura-red.html (accessed
    September 25, 2010).

18. "Natural Red Food Color." Nature's Flavors. naturesflavors.com
    /product_info.php?cPath=72&products_id=3369 (accessed Septem-
    ber 25, 2010).

19. "Health Evaluation Fact Sheet — Toluene." California Dept. of Health
    Services. cdph.ca.gov/programs/hesis/Documents/toluene.pdf (ac-
    cessed July 12, 2011).

20. Environmental Health Association of Nova Scotia. "Why No Synthetic
    Fragrances?" Guide to Less Toxic Products. lesstoxicguide.ca/index.asp
    ?fetch=usage#synethetic (accessed October 12, 2010).

21. Sanofi Pasteur. "Fluzone Prescribing Information." Vaccine Information
    Shoppe. vaccineshoppe.com/image.cfm?image_type=product_pdf
    π=flu (accessed September 10, 2010).

22. Thompson, William, Cristofer Price, Barbara Goodson et al. "Early
    Thimerosal Exposure and Neuropsychological Outcomes at 7 to 10
    Years." *The New England Journal of Medicine.* nejm.org/doi/full/10.1056
    /NEJMoa071434 (accessed July 13, 2011).

23. Medscape.medscape.com/viewarticle/727881 (accessed September 10,
    2010).

Part 3: The Baseline

1. EWG, Campaign for Safe Cosmetics. "Not So Sexy: Hidden Chemicals in Perfume and Colognes." Environmental Working Group. ewg .org/notsosexy (accessed September 18, 2010).

2. "Chanel Paradoxal Nail Polish: Fall's It Shade." Adventures in the Stiletto Jungle. stilettojungleblog.com/2010/08/chanel-paradoxal-nail -polish-falls-it.html (accessed September 14, 2010).

3. "List of nail products containing DBP." Environmental Working Group. ewg.org/node/8164 (accessed September 15, 2010).

4. National Cancer Institute. "Antiperspirants/Deodorants and Breast Cancer." Comprehensive Cancer Information. cancer.gov/cancertopics /factsheet/Risk/AP-Deo (accessed September 2, 2010).

5. Seattle Public Utilities. "Cedar Tolt Water Quality." City of Seattle. cityofseattle.net/util/groups/public/@spu/@ssw/documents/web content/substances_200312020913218.pdf (accessed September 5, 2010).

6. City of Seattle. "Seattle Public Utilities — Water Quality." The Official Web Site for the City of Seattle, Washington. cityofseattle.net/util /Services/Water/Water_Quality/LEAD_200312011625223.asp (accessed September 22, 2010).

7. "Testing Services for Private Wells." Anatek Labs, Inc. anateklabs.com /pages/default.asp?PageTextID=19 (accessed September 10, 2010).

8. Shabecoff, Philip and Alice Shabecoff. *Poisoned Profits: The Toxic Assault on Our Children*. New York: Random House, 2008.

9. Fitzgerald, Randall. *The Hundred-Year Lie: How to Protect Yourself from the Chemicals That Are Destroying Your Health*. New York: Plume, 2007.

10. Fitzgerald, Randall. *The Hundred-Year Lie: How to Protect Yourself from the Chemicals That Are Destroying Your Health*. New York: Plume, 2007.

11. Ginsberg, Gary and Brian Toal. *What's Toxic, What's Not*. Berkley trade paperback ed. New York: Berkley Books, 2006.

12. Fitzgerald, Randall. *The Hundred-Year Lie: How to Protect Yourself from the Chemicals That Are Destroying Your Health*. New York: Plume, 2007.

13. Shabecoff, Philip and Alice Shabecoff. *Poisoned Profits: The Toxic Assault on Our Children*. New York: Random House, 2008.

14. Fitzgerald, Randall. *The Hundred-Year Lie: How to Protect Yourself from the Chemicals That Are Destroying Your Health*. New York: Plume, 2007.

15. Fitzgerald, Randall. *The Hundred-Year Lie: How to Protect Yourself from the Chemicals That Are Destroying Your Health*. New York: Plume, 2007.

16. "Take Back Your Meds." Take Back Your Meds. medicinereturn.com (accessed September 15, 2010).

17. "EcoFlo Family Water Pitcher." EcoFlo. ecoflowater.com/store/family-water-pitcher/flypage.tpl.html (accessed September 15, 2010).

18. Raver, Anne. "Need an Air Freshener? Try Plants." *The New York Times*. query.nytimes.com/gst/fullpage.html?res=9C0CE7DD1138F930A257 51C0A962958260&sec=&spon=&pagewanted=all (accessed October 22, 2010).

19. "The Best Houseplants for a Healthy Home." HGTV Canada. hgtv.ca/gardening/articledetails.aspx?ContentId=800&cat=2&by=10 (accessed October 22, 2010).

20. "The Best Houseplants for a Healthy Home." HGTV Canada. hgtv.ca/gardening/articledetails.aspx?ContentId=800&cat=2&by=10 (accessed October 22, 2010).

21. Raver, Anne. "Need an Air Freshener? Try Plants." *The New York Times*. query.nytimes.com/gst/fullpage.html?res=9C0CE7DD1138F930A257 51C0A962958260&sec=&spon=&pagewanted=all (accessed October 22, 2010).

22. "15 houseplants for improving indoor air quality." Mother Nature Network. mnn.com/your-home/green-building-remodeling/photos/15-houseplants-for-improving-indoor-air-quality (accessed October 22, 2010).

23. "Best Plants for Indoor Air Quality." The Daily Green. thedailygreen.com/going-green/tips/best-plants-for-indoor-air-quality (accessed October 22, 2010).

24. "Top 10 Natural, Eco-Friendly and Anti-Pollutant Houseplants." The New Ecologist. thenewecologist.com/2009/07/top-10-natural-eco-friendly-and-anti-pollutant-houseplants/ (accessed October 22, 2010).

25. Shapley, Dan. "Plants and VOCs." The Daily Green. thedailygreen.com/environmental-news/latest/house-plants-vocs-47090401 (accessed October 22, 2010).

26. Grady, Denise. "First Signs of Puberty Seen in Younger Girls." *The New York Times*. nytimes.com/2010/08/09/health/research/09puberty.html (accessed October 22, 2010).

27. "Pubertal Assessment Method and Baseline Characteristics in a Mixed Longitudinal Study of Girls." Pediatrics | Official Journal of the American Academy of Pediatrics. pediatrics.aappublications.org/cgi/content/abstract/peds.2009-3079v1 (accessed October 31, 2010).

28. "Is BPA Making Our Kids Grow Up Faster?" Washington Toxics Coalition. watoxics.org/toxicswatch/is-bpa-making-our-kids-grow-up-faster (accessed October 31, 2010).

29. "Is BPA Making Our Kids Grow Up Faster?" Washington Toxics Co-

alition. watoxics.org/toxicswatch/is-bpa-making-our-kids-grow-up
-faster (accessed October 31, 2010).

30. "Recent Findings on Early Puberty in Girls Highlight Urgent Need
for New Chemicals Policy." Safer Chemicals, Healthy Families. safer
chemicals.org/2010/08/recent-findings-on-early-puberty-in-girls-high
light-urgent-need-for-new-chemicals-policy.html (accessed October 31,
2010).

31. "Tips to Green Your Halloween." Environmental Working Group.
ewg.org/healthyhometips/halloweentips?utm_source=halloweenfull
&utm_medium=email&utm_content=first-link&utm_campaign=hht
(accessed October 31, 2010).

32. "PFC—Perfluorinated Chemicals." Sailhome. sailhome.org/Concerns
/BodyBurden/Burdens/PFC.html (accessed November 10, 2010).

33. "DenTek Floss." DenTek Oral Care. dentek.com/store/index.php?
dispatch=categories.view&category_id=39 (accessed November 10,
2010).

34. "PFCs: Stain-Resistant Teflon Chemicals." Alliance for a Clean and
Healthy Maine. cleanandhealthyme.org/BodyofEvidenceReport/The
Chemicals/PFCsStainResistantTeflonChemicals/tabid/98/Default
.aspx (accessed November 10, 2010).

35. Sefton, Dru. "You wouldn't believe what lives in your pillows." *The
Seattle Times*. seattletimes.nwsource.com/html/health/2002632280
_healthpillows20.html (accessed November 25, 2010).

36. Sherbenou, Ed. "Haz-Mat: Tempur-Pedic Memory Foam Mattress
Outgassing?" Air Purifier Reviews and Purification Technology Reports. air-purifier-power.com/tempurpedicmemoryfoammatresstoxic
013010.html (accessed November 25, 2010).

37. Price, Trevor. "High Level Evaluation of Tempurpedic Beds." Article Alley.
articlealley.com/article_704685_47.html (accessed November 30, 2010).

38. "Safety of Tempur-Pedic Mattresses." eHow. ehow.com/facts_5927643
_safety-tempur_pedic-mattresses.html (accessed November 30, 2010).

39. Greenhalgh, Jane. "Blowing the Whistle On 'Brazilian Blowout' Hair
Straightener." NPR : National Public Radio . npr.org/templates/story
/story.php?storyId=130667357 (accessed December 5, 2010).

40. "Brazilian Blowout Solution contains formaldehyde." Health Canada.
hc-sc.gc.ca/ahc-asc/media/advisories-avis/_2010/2010_167-eng.php
(accessed December 5, 2010).

41. "Testing Your Home For Lead." Environmental Protection Agency.
epa.gov/lead/pubs/leadtest.pdf (accessed December 5, 2010).

42. "Human Toxome Project—Diethyl phthalate." Environmental Working

Group. ewg.org/sites/humantoxome/chemicals/chemical.php
?chemid=70002 (accessed December 15, 2010).

43. "Human Toxome Project—Monoethyl phthalate." Environmental
Working Group. ewg.org/sites/humantoxome/chemicals/chemical
.php?chemid=100364 (accessed December 15, 2010).

44. "Human Toxome Project—Mono-(2-ethyl-5-hydroxyhexyl) phthalate." Environmental Working Group. ewg.org/sites/humantoxome/
chemicals/chemical.php?chemid=100360 (accessed December 15, 2010).

45. "Human Toxome Project—Mono-(2-ethyl-5-hydroxyhexyl) phthalate." Environmental Working Group. ewg.org/sites/humantoxome/
chemicals/chemical.php?chemid=100360 (accessed December 15, 2010).

46. "Human Toxome Project—Mono-(2-ethyl-5-oxohexyl) phthalate." Environmental Working Group. ewg.org/sites/humantoxome/chemicals
/chemical.php?chemid=100361 (accessed December 15, 2010).

47. "Human Toxome Project—Propylparaben." Environmental Working
Group. ewg.org/sites/humantoxome/chemicals/chemical.php?chemid
=90007 (accessed December 15, 2010).

48. "Human Toxome Project—Propylparaben." Environmental Working
Group. ewg.org/sites/humantoxome/chemicals/chemical.php?chemid
=90007 (accessed December 15, 2010).

49. "Human Toxome Project—Methylparaben." Environmental Working
Group. ewg.org/sites/humantoxome/chemicals/chemical.php?chemid
=90004 (accessed December 15, 2010).

50. "Human Toxome Project—Methylparaben." Environmental Working
Group. ewg.org/sites/humantoxome/chemicals/chemical.php?chemid
=90004 (accessed December 15, 2010).

51. "Human Toxome Project—Ethylparaben." Environmental Working
Group. ewg.org/sites/humantoxome/chemicals/chemical.php?chemid
=90005 (accessed December 15, 2010).

52. "Human Toxome Project—Butylparaben." Environmental Working
Group. ewg.org/sites/humantoxome/chemicals/chemical.php?chemid
=90008 (accessed December 15, 2010).

53. "Hawaiian Tropic Sensitive Skin Face Lotion Sunscreen, SPF 30."
Skin Deep: Cosmetic Safety Reviews. cosmeticdatabase.com/product
/320748/Hawaiian_Tropic_Sensitive_Skin_Face_Lotion_Sunscreen
%2C_SPF_30/ (accessed December 20, 2010).

54. Enersen, Jean. "Chemicals complicate Halloween costume shopping."
KING 5 News. king5.com/health/59758232.html (accessed November
10, 2010).

55. "Desert Commando Camo Child Costume." Halloween Costumes.

spirithalloween.com/product/desert-commando-camo-child-costume-/
(accessed November 13, 2010).

56. "Molybdenum information page." Zest for Life. anyvitamins.com/moly
bdenum-info.htm (accessed December 17, 2010).

57. "Human Toxome Project — Arsenic." Environmental Working Group.
ewg.org/sites/humantoxome/chemicals/chemical.php?chemid=30003
(accessed December 28, 2010).

58. "Human Toxome Project — Lead." Environmental Working Group.
ewg.org/sites/humantoxome/chemicals/chemical.php?chemid=30001
(accessed December 28, 2010).

59. "Human Toxome Project — Mercury." Environmental Working Group.
ewg.org/sites/humantoxome/chemicals/chemical.php?chemid=100375
(accessed December 28, 2010).

60. "Human Toxome Project — Mercury." Environmental Working Group.
ewg.org/sites/humantoxome/chemicals/chemical.php?chemid=100375
(accessed December 28, 2010).

61. "Human Toxome Project — Mercury." Environmental Working Group.
ewg.org/sites/humantoxome/chemicals/chemical.php?chemid=100375
(accessed December 28, 2010).

62. Morrissey, Michael, Rosalee Rasmussen and Tomoko Okada. "Mercury
Content in Pacific Troll-Caught." NOAA: National Marine Fisheries
Service. nmfs.noaa.gov/fishwatch/docs/OSU_Mercury_Study.pdf (ac-
cessed December 11, 2010).

Part 4: Adjusting to Non-Toxic Living

1. Hanson, David J. "Alcohol And Health." State University of New York.
www2.potsdam.edu/hansondj/AlcoholAndHealth.html (accessed July
14, 2011).

2. "Organic Wines and Sulfites." Organic Wine Company. ecowine.com
/sulfites.htm (accessed December 29, 2010).

3. "Study: Pesticides found in wine." PhysOrg.com — Science News, Technology, Physics. physorg.com/news126540989.html (accessed December 29, 2010).

4. "Home Heating Fuel Oil Spills." Wisconsin Department of Health
Services. dhs.wisconsin.gov/eh/air/fs/Oilspill.htm (accessed December 29, 2010).

5. "Heating methods and open burning." Canadian Lung Association.
lung.ca/protect-protegez/pollution-pollution/outdoor-exterior/heating
-chauffage_e.php (accessed December 29, 2010).

6. "Soaps & Detergent: (1900s to Now)." The American Cleaning Institute.

cleaninginstitute.org/clean_living/soaps__detergent_history_3.aspx (accessed December 12, 2010).

7. Fauteux, Ray. "Bar soap vs. body wash." Helium. helium.com/items /822985-bar-soap-vs-body-wash (accessed December 7, 2010).

8. Newman, Andrew Adam. "Adding a Masculine Edge to Body Wash." *The New York Times*. nytimes.com/2009/09/08/business/media/08a dco.html (accessed December 7, 2010).

9. "Women's Purchasing Power Grows" RetailWire. retailwire.com /Discussions/Sngl_Discussion.cfm/13569 (accessed December 7, 2010).

10. Newman, Andrew Adam. "Adding a Masculine Edge to Body Wash." *The New York Times*. nytimes.com/2009/09/08/business/media/08a dco.html (accessed December 7, 2010).

11. Simmons, Sunshine. "Bar soap vs. body wash." Helium. helium.com /items/829811-bar-soap-vs-body-wash (accessed December 22, 2010).

12. "Certain Dri Antiperspirant Roll-On." Skin Deep: Cosmetic Safety Reviews. cosmeticdatabase.com/product/216951/Certain_Dri_Anti perspirant_Roll-On/ (accessed December 7, 2010).

13. "Murad Acne Body Wash." Skin Deep: Cosmetic Safety Reviews. cosmeticdatabase.com/product/154117/Murad_Acne_Body_Wash/ (accessed January 15, 2011).

14. "Resorcinol." Skin Deep: Cosmetic Safety Reviews. cosmeticsdatabase .com/ingredient/705539/RESORCINOL/ (accessed January 15, 2011).

15. Aggarwal, Bharat. "Anticancer Potential of Curcumin." M. D. Anderson Cancer Center. houston.myeloma.org/Tumeric.pdf (accessed December 15, 2010).

16. "Sunscreens Exposed: 9 surprising truths." Environmental Working Group. ewg.org/2010sunscreen/9-surprising-facts-about-sunscreen/ (accessed December 22, 2010).

17. "EWG's 2010 Sunscreen Guide." Environmental Working Group. ewg.org/2010sunscreen/faqs-2010/#question_30 (accessed December 22, 2010).

18. "HDPE (High Density Polyethylene) Pipe." Build It Green. buildit green.org/attachments/wysiwyg/22/HDPE-Pipe.pdf (accessed November 15, 2010).

19. Dickey, Philip. "Keeping Molehills from Becoming Mountains." Washington Toxics Coalition. watoxics.org/files/moles.pdf (accessed December 30, 2010).

20. Ritter, Stephen K. "Exposure Routes Confound BPA Debate." American Chemical Society Publications. pubs.acs.org/cen/coverstory/89 /8923cover3.html (accessed July 14, 2011).

21. "Guide to Less Toxic Products." Environmental Health Association of Nova Scotia. lesstoxicguide.ca/ (accessed December 22, 2010).

Part 5: Going a Little Bit Bonkers

1. Gavigan, Christopher. "Beware of Lead in Christmas Trees and Lights." Healthy Child Healthy World. healthychild.org/blog/comments/tip _79_beware_of_lead_in_christmas_trees_and_lights/ (accessed December 8, 2010).

2. Ajda, G., A. Thansandote, E. Lemay, J. McNamee and P. V. Bellier. "Estimation of Ambient Electric Fields Generated by Dirty Electricity from Compact Fluorescent Lamps." Health Canada. bioelectromagnet ics.org/bems2010/supp_data/P-B-134.pdf (accessed December 17, 2010).

3. Weeks, Brad. "Just say NO to compact fluorescent bulbs." The Weeks Clinic for Corrective Medicine and Psychiatry. weeksmd.com/?p=899 (accessed July 14, 2011).

4. Segell, Michael. "11 Ways to Protect Yourself from Dirty Electricity." *Prevention Magazine*. prevention.com/electroshocker/index.shtml (accessed December 22, 2010).

5. "Is My Cell Phone Dangerous?" Environmental Working Group. ewg .org/cellphoneradiation/8-Safety-Tips (accessed December 22, 2010).

6. "Enteric coating." Wikipedia. en.wikipedia.org/wiki/Enteric_coating (accessed January 2, 2011).

7. "Ecover Dishwasher Tablets, Material Safety Data Sheet." Ecover. ecover .com/NR/rdonlyres/20046BE0-F78F-413B-B522-59139D561618/5197 /MSDS.pdf (accessed January 2, 2011).

8. "Emission and Residue Characteristics from Burning Artificial Wax Firelogs." Environmental Protection Agency. epa.gov/ttn/chief/con ference/ei15/poster/li_poster.pdf (accessed December 29, 2010).

9. "Where is PVC, the Poison Plastic Hiding in Your School?" BE SAFE Precautionary Campaign. besafenet.com/pvc/thisvinylschool/ (accessed October 1, 2010).

10. MacIntosh, Helen Suh. "Are Tattoo Inks Toxic?" TreeHugger. tree hugger.com/files/2007/04/tattoo_inks_toxic.php (accessed October 4, 2010).

11. "Green Tattoo Removal Process." Good Chemistry. good-chemistry.org /?p=1434 (accessed October 5, 2010).

12. "Think Before You Ink: Are Tattoos Safe?" U.S. Food and Drug Administration. fda.gov/ForConsumers/ConsumerUpdates/ucm048919. htm (accessed October 7, 2010).

13. Healy, Bernadine. "The Dangerous Art of the Tattoo." U.S. News and

World Report. health.usnews.com/health-news/family-health/articles
/2008/07/25/the-dangerous-art-of-the-tattoo.html (accessed October
5, 2010).

14. "Think Before You Ink: Are Tattoos Safe?" U.S. Food and Drug Administration. fda.gov/downloads/ForConsumers/ConsumerUpdates/
UCM143401.pdf (accessed October 6, 2010).

15. "Chlorinated Pesticide Exposure Testing." Metametrix Clinical Laboratory. metametrix.com/test-menu/profiles/toxicants-and-detoxification
/chlorinated-pesticide-exposure-testing (accessed November 17, 2010).

16. "Polychlorinated Biphenyl Testing for Body Burden." Metametrix Clinical Laboratory. metametrix.com/test-menu/profiles/toxicants-and
-detoxification/polychlorinated-biphenyl-testing?t=overview (accessed
November 17, 2010).

17. "Volatile Solvent Test." Metametrix Clinical Laboratory. metametrix
.com/test-menu/profiles/toxicants-and-detoxification/volatile-solvents
?t=overview (accessed November 17, 2010).

18. Striepe, Becky. "Pomi Tomatoes: A BPA Free Alternative to Cans." Eat
Drink Better. eatdrinkbetter.com/2010/06/23/pomi-tomatoes-a-bpa
-free-alternative-to-cans/ (accessed December 16, 2010).

19. Scoleri, Kathy. "General Mills Muir Glen Ditching BPA in Canned
Tomatoes." SafeMama. safemama.com/2010/11/03/general-mills-muir
-glen-ditching-bpa-in-canned-tomatoes-but/ (accessed December 17,
2010).

20. "BPA is Invading Your Wallet!" Washington Toxics Coalition. watoxics
.org/toxicswatch/bpa-is-invading-your-wallet (accessed December 29,
2010).

21. Connor, Siobhan and Alexandra Spunt. *No More Dirty Looks: The
Truth About Your Beauty Products — and the Ultimate Guide to Safe and
Clean Cosmetics.* New York: Da Capo Lifelong, 2010.

Part 6: Figuring It All Out

1. Zissu, Alexandra. "Safe Organic Hair Dye Products — Non-toxic Organic Hair Dyes." The Daily Green. thedailygreen.com/living-green
/blogs/organic-parenting/non-toxic-hair-dyes-55021302 (accessed
July 15, 2011).

2. Connor, Siobhan and Alexandra Spunt. *No More Dirty Looks: The
Truth About Your Beauty Products — and the Ultimate Guide to Safe and
Clean Cosmetics.* New York: Da Capo Lifelong, 2010.

3. Environmental Working Group. "Cosmetic Safety Database." Skin
Deep. cosmeticdatabase.com/ (accessed February 22, 2011).

4. "15-inch MacBook Pro Environmental Report." Apple. images.apple

.com/environment/reports/docs/MacBook-Pro-15-inch-Environmental
-Report_April2010.pdf (accessed December 17, 2010).

5. Fitzgerald, Randall. *The Hundred-Year Lie: How to Protect Yourself from
the Chemicals That Are Destroying Your Health.* Plume, 2006.

6. Kay, Jane. "Hazard warning on home cleaners." Featured Articles. articles
.sfgate.com/2007-07-24/news/17252262_1_toxic-chemicals-cleaning
-products-research-group (accessed October 15, 2010).

7. HealthyStuff.org. "Rating System for Toys." Researching Toxic Chemicals in Everyday Products. healthystuff.org/departments/toys/about
.ranking.php (accessed March 1, 2011).

Index

If you have enjoyed *The Non-Toxic Avenger*, you might also enjoy other

BOOKS TO BUILD A NEW SOCIETY

Our books provide positive solutions for people who want to make a difference. We specialize in:

Sustainable Living • Green Building • Peak Oil
Renewable Energy • Environment & Economy
Natural Building & Appropriate Technology
Progressive Leadership • Resistance and Community
Educational & Parenting Resources

New Society Publishers

ENVIRONMENTAL BENEFITS STATEMENT

New Society Publishers has chosen to produce this book on recycled paper made with **100% post consumer waste,** processed chlorine free, and old growth free.

For every 5,000 books printed, New Society saves the following resources:[1]

29	Trees
2,604	Pounds of Solid Waste
2,865	Gallons of Water
3,737	Kilowatt Hours of Electricity
4,734	Pounds of Greenhouse Gases
20	Pounds of HAPs, VOCs, and AOX Combined
7	Cubic Yards of Landfill Space

[1]Environmental benefits are calculated based on research done by the Environmental Defense Fund and other members of the Paper Task Force who study the environmental impacts of the paper industry.

For a full list of NSP's titles, please call 1-800-567-6772 or check out our website at:

www.newsociety.com

NEW SOCIETY PUBLISHERS

About the Author

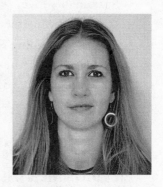

Deanna Duke lives in Seattle with her husband and two children and writes the highly read environmental blog, *The Crunchy Chicken* (www.the crunchychicken.com). The focus of her work is in educating others on environmental issues and explaining how she and her family have not only lowered their carbon footprint and impact on the environment, but also reduced their exposure to toxic chemicals in their home, work and school environments.

By day, Deanna works for a regional governmental natural resources agency. In addition to her blog, she also writes as an Expert Urban Homesteader for *Mother Earth News Online* and is the Personal Care Consultant for the eco-makeover television show, *Mission: Sustainable*.

Deanna is regularly interviewed as a green expert by major media outlets such as *The New York Times*, *USA Today*, *The Scientific American* and the *National Enquirer*. Technorati has listed her blog in the top 3,000 blogs (out of 3 million) and her monthly imprints average around 50,000.